Curing Madness

By Jason Pegler

The Selected Works of a former manic depressive

"To cure a mental illness is always possible. If you always believe so it will happen. This is how I transformed myself. You too can do the same if you decide to do so". Jason Pegler

Published by
Chipmunkapublishing
PO Box 6872
Brentwood
Essex CM13 1ZT
United Kingdom

First published 2006

Contact the author: jasonpegler@yahoo.com

A record of this book is in the British Library.

http://www.chipmunkapublishing.com

CONTENTS

"To cure a mental illness is always possible. If you always believe so it will happen. This is how I transformed myself. You too can do the same if you decide to do so".

Jason Pegler 2006

DEDICATION

I want to dedicate this book to Alistair Priestly who I went to school with who so sadly took his own life recently, his family and his friends. I would also like to dedicate this book to my girlfriend, my friends and family who have stuck by me through thick and thin. You have helped provide me with the strength to lead a life in which I am fortunate to be able to focus on my goals to help empower people who have suffered from mental health issues. I would not feel that this book had any real accuracy or value though, unless I thank one man in particular. That man is a man who I have shaken hands with twice just before walking on fire: the American life coach, Anthony Robbins. From the year 2000 I started reading Anthony Robbins' books and found his work inspiring. By studying his material and applying it to my own life I managed to gain more and more internal strength and my inner voice grew. In September 2004 I finally met him at one of his Power Seminars and it was during these days that I finally decided to come off the psychiatric medication. By the end of 2004 I managed to come off whilst liaising with my psychiatrist and to my delight I have never looked back. My life has improved dramatically since this time and I know I will never be back on this medication or in a mental hospital again, unless I am visiting with the intention of meeting patients and improving the way the services are run.

Ever since this moment I felt motivated to carry on with 'Curing Madness' and as I come to realise the end of this project my cure is complete. This release of positive chi now gives me new found strength to continue dedicating my life, and the life of others, through my work with Chipmunkapublishing the

Chipmunka Group and related companies, to harness the largest civil rights movement of all time. Giving a voice to those with "mental health issues", so we can prevent the suffering, humiliation, injustice and abuse that these people and their friends and families sometimes face.

INTRODUCTION

I am now completely free from the psychiatric drugs that I took from the ages of 17 to 29. I am fortunate that I have been able to rebuild my life and lead a full recovery so I could come off the medication and never look back. I believe that no matter how mentally ill someone becomes that they can cure themselves if they choose to do so and take steps every day. Read this book first and then re-evaluate your life, find out what your values are and work out your diet, physical exercise and emotional intelligence. Take appropriate advice and then there is no reason why you can't get off completely recover and lead a fantastic life using the pain you once had to help other people in the world.

This book has some real challenges ahead. If I slip into utopian mode please bear with me, such is the nature of a former manic depressive. The mission of this book is to focus on saving the world from itself, most notably to stop the humiliation and stigma of the "mentally ill" and to prove that practising NLP and harnessing creativity really can work and form the basis of new and improved mental health services. I believe that if new techniques are used appropriately and at first point of contact with patients that there will be no need for psychiatry or drug companies to play any roles in the mental health or well being industry.

Curing madness is the follow up to my autobiography on living with manic depression, A Can of Madness. A Can of Madness is a rollercoaster ride about coming to terms with living with manic depression and making a 90% recovery. It has helped thousands of people realise that they are not the only person in the world, that they go through such amazing highs and lows and enables loved ones to finally see and understand what their partners, friends and family are going through. However, this is still not enough.

Everyday more and more people are being falsely diagnosed with mental illness for life and being over medicated at the hands of governments and the drug companies. There needs to be a global shift in communication in the "mental health world" as Martin Luther King did for black rights and Bob Geldof did for Africa.

By writing Curing Madness I am making my personal testimony as a social entrepreneur, rap artist, consultant, publisher, speaker, Chief Executive and Chairman to prove that I was able to cure myself by taking consistent positives steps, and taking massive action. By believing I could get better I actually did. It is my view that anyone who has ever been diagnosed with a mental illness can do the same thing and my duty as a human being to create a system and work with other like minded people who share this vision and are capable of doing something about it.

For me writing Curing Madness is the next step. It is a quantum leap from my previous book. A Can of Madness was said by the Big Issue to make Prozac Nation look like a walk in the park. I hope from the deepest part of my soul that Curing Madness will demonstrate that anything in life is possible no matter what your previous psychiatric or social history.

There are two hurdles to overcome. Firstly, pill popping is now so prevalent in our culture that it is already an epidemic. This action must be replaced by looking for alternative therapies; most notably people must be given the best tools such as practising NLP, hypnosis and being encouraged to raise their self esteem and expectations of their own lives. The great work of practitioners like Anthony Robbins and Paul McKenna must be brought inside systems such as schools and the NHS. We must go a stage further with Robbins and McKenna in future generations and make the services they practise free across society so that these systems are intertwined into our culture. I believe passionately that the work that I am doing is central in achieving this purpose. History will tell us the answer.

Secondly, there has been thousands of years of psychological and now psychiatric oppression in most places on the planet and people who are different or have mental health issues have never had a voice. By using my own personal testimony I make myself an example of how the world is changing in this regard and how people have moved from their own disempowered self to thinking and empowering others.

My mission is a utopian one and can best be understood by studying the diagram below.

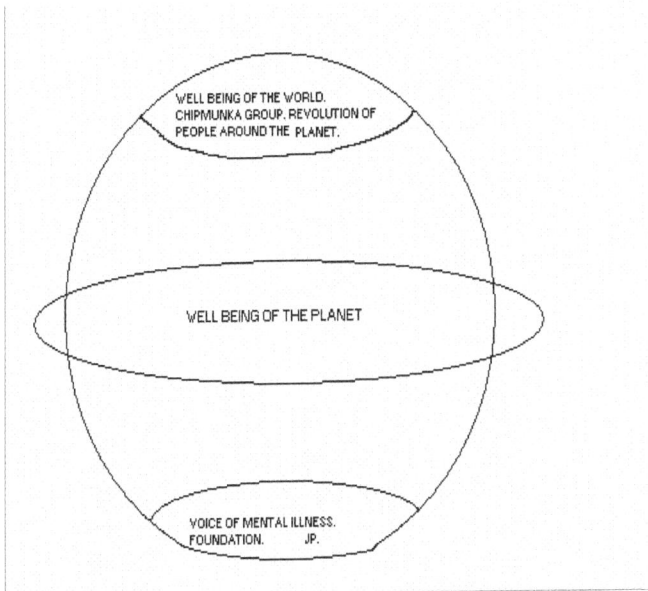

Figure 1.1

The diagram above illustrates how I can achieve my utopian goal. My main work goal in life is to reduce the humiliation of people with mental illness. I visualize this goal working so I can place it in the well being section in the diagram above. To achieve my goal I use a variety of steps. At the bottom of the diagram I put in the small steps. For example, in this section I would include the Chipmunka Foundation (see www.chipmunkafoundation.org: Registered charity number 1109537). The fact we help people with mental illness and the fact that I as an individual have had manic depression and recovered from it gives me a passion for wanting to work in this area.

In my view the steps at the bottom of figure 1.1 are necessary steps towards the utopian goal. The big steps would be the Chipmunka Group, including Chipmunkapublishing. The fact that I set up Chipmunkapublishing as the Mental Health Publisher enabled me to set up the Chipmunka Foundation. Even if the Chipmunka Foundation achieves its mission and becomes the most effective and significant mental health charity in the world it will not become a bigger influence than Chipmunkapublishing or the Chipmunka Group as they were the catalyst for it.

The Chipmunka Group is a social entrepreneurship and philanthropic model that enables the Foundation to grow organically. Resources from the Group "The World's first Mental Health brand" are pumped into the Foundation. The Chipmunka Group generates its own revenue.....and actively supports the Foundation. It also gives opportunities to people with mental health issues to become self-employed, social entrepreneurs and show that people with mental health issues can achieve anything that they believe is possible therefore creating the world's first mental health celebrities.

The charity in itself, although it can transcend economies in a humanitarian context does not in an economic, political or socioeconomic sense.

The Chipmunka Group itself has the same mission as the Foundation but uses economic forces to take a bigger step. Therefore, all parts of the Chipmunka Group would go above the goal cylinder because of their economic potential.

The fact that my life's mission is to help people with mental illness is also in my eyes a small step. By October 2005 Chipmunkapublishing alone receives more web traffic than any other mental health organization in UK with over 15,000 visitors every week. This is because we are giving people a voice, an opportunity to have their voices heard in a world where they are discriminated against.

The reason why I have put helping people with mental illness as a small step is simple. I deliberately used the wrong language. There is no such thing as mental illness really[1]. For mental illness is a mindset, i.e. something that is self manifested. If you decide you wil get better then you will. This is something that can only come from within and why NLP should be used to conquer it. Mental illness is also a manufactured term set up as a form of social control as governments do not generally want people to think for themselves. The drug companies also always have vested interest as their goal is to make a profit out of their products and influence psychiatry and governments worldwide to increase the profits of their shareholders like any other business.

The big step in Figure 1.1 is to improve the well being of people on the planet. The real voice here is changing the term mental illness and turning it into well being. If people see the issue as well being there will be no taboo. They will realize that mental illness affects everyone. Then they will be more inclined to talk about mental health and then more likely to help a homeless person when they see one and not just give them a handout that will more than likely be spent on drugs,

[1] For further reading read "The Necessity of Madness by John Breeding published by Chipmunkapublishing.

but talk to them or give them an opportunity to get employed and manage their own life or money or offer them appropriate support[2].

The other advantage of using well being is also the mindset of the person with the "mental health issue." They will see their state as something that can be felt by more people or even anyone.

Then they can see a way out, change their mindset and cure themselves. With this paradigm shift[3] the drug companies and psychiatrists influence on the world will lessen, their grips will loosen and new well being ......will be developed creating a healthier happier world.

The final small step I would like to discuss is the fact that I as a former manic depressive have legitimacy in the area of "reducing the humiliation of people with mental illness" because I am one of the many people who have actually experienced it and not merely observed it.

By the time I'd set up Chipmunkapublishing in April 2002 and launched my autobiography on living with manic depression "A Can of Madness". I knew that my story was an example of someone who was prepared to face up to what being diagnosed with a mental illness meant in the eyes of society. In fact what motivated me to write it was to stop the humiliation and suffering of another 17 year old with manic depression.

---

[2] The Big Issue set up in 1991 to empower homeless people has pioneered this social phenomenon.
[3] 'paradigm shift' a term used by Stephen R Covey author of The 7 habits of Highly Effective People.

This is because I went through it first when I was 17 and it is only natural to want to stop someone else going through the same point that you went through. This is a natural human instinct. I am no different than any other human being. This is precisely why my own experience is a small step in the universe. My experience planted the seeds for Chipmunkapublishing, the Chipmunka Group and the Foundation and is my driving force for realising my goal to eliminate global humiliation. It is my passion that makes me get up buzzing every day and commit more and shapes my belief systems and well being. I am only one person.

The goal many of us have is to stop the humiliation of anyone who has been told they have a mental illness because this is an ideal. It is something that in our eyes should not occur in the 21st Century or should have ever occurred in history. This is a utopian goal but one that a growing number of us believe is possible. The big step here would be a crowd of people stepping out as we have done and using mental health as a positive thus creating a paradigm shift. This would require millions of people stepping up around the world and saying why the humiliation of mental illness is wrong. This like anything only receives real credibility and revolutionary status if it is led and controlled by the "sufferers" themselves, by the people who went through it. The goal is beyond our egos, it's beyond the Chipmunka Group and beyond the thousands of mental health charities and service user groups around the world. It's about millions of people all around the world being brave enough to stand up for what they believe as human beings and having the mental strength to give back and take on the responsibility of giving others an opportunity to empower themselves for the well being of the world and the planet. This is for all of our sakes; for the future well being of everyone on the planet; for our children and our children's children, for people in the 3rd world, so we live on a humanitarian world. So we can live in a world of peace and a world without global warming.

Let's go into more detail about the Brand. A brand is needed to bring all this to the public domain. When I set up Chipmunkapublishing it was a great idea but just the first thing that happened. Let me explain by talking about my own experiences. When I was 17 I had been in a mental hospital for six weeks[4], thinking that I was god and that my life was football manager the computer game. Typical of feeling high you may say. From the age of 17 when I came down from mania I had an epiphany. The moment I became aware I was living in a mental hospital I had a shocking feeling of humiliation and guilt in my heart, body and soul. Humiliation that all those realisations I had were not true in the "real world" and guilt that I couldn't have cared less about people who were in 'mental institutions' until I was actually in one myself. Immediately I had a life long mission. The first was to make a Hollywood blockbuster movie about my own life to explain the previously unimaginable humiliation that I felt, because this was the only way that I would ever psychoanalyse myself and heal 100%. Secondly, I now had a new insight into the pain, humiliation and suffering of others and I wanted to stop another 17 year old from going through the same pain and indeed anyone else that I could possibly help.

---

[4] This was the first of 5 psychiatric admissions between 1993 and 2000.

So, writing and Publishing were the first things that happened in the public domain. Now there are so many things going on that I am actually creating the world's first mental health brand. When you think of Computer Software you think of Microsoft, when you think of Music you think of Sony, when you think of mental health and want you to think of well being instead and then think of Chipmunka or come up with something amazing and people will support that too. You can use NLP techniques, honesty, marketing; it doesn't matter as long as your intentions are true to yourself and you feel comfortable with it. Being diagnosed with manic depression made me more sensitive as a human being and gave me the opportunity to make a choice, and I chose to help other people. It's a natural response and is, I believe, an example of the humanitarian nature in all of us.

So with the economic and humanitarian models working in tandem the charity and social corporate models have the opportunity to squeeze together and create this utopia. This is the mission. Let's see what's been happening over the last few years and draw some inspiration first before we get to the nuts and bolts later on.

Well, since 1969 there has been a campaign led by the Citizens Campaign for Human Rights to kill psychiatry. An interesting aim, supported by Scientologists worldwide, including Tom Cruise and John Travolta. I have a lot of sympathy with their view as they report the truth but they fail to provide the ultimate alternative that will replace psychiatry when they aim to dethrone it by 2010. They attack psychiatrists head on as they have blood on their hands, because the drugs companies that so cleverly force the world to take drugs for their own gain are too hard to dismantle without taking away their foundation i.e. the drug pushers and sellers, the psychiatrists. This is certainly a hard liners views and I believe necessary for someone to be taking an anti psychiatry stance because it has such a massive influence on the mental health system as the device used by the drug companies to sell their products. Mr Hubbard would be naïve not to be aware that no matter how successful he believed his work would become that an organisation cannot change the world, nor can an individual. It is the people within it that shape what happens in the world. The rise of the madman is inevitable. My mission in life is to facilitate the empowerment of the madman in the most forceful way that I can. Then more lives can be saved and we will all accept openly that we are all a little bit crazy.

We are convinced that the rise of the mental health sufferer is the biggest civil rights movement of all time. This could also be described as a social evolution. The social evolution that is taking place we believe is more important than mass world communication, terrorism and third world debt together. I believe that if everyone in the world was mentally well that none of these problems would exist. There would be no need for them to exist. More and more people are becoming aware of this. By 2050 the humiliation that mental illness brings will have disappeared. Then the one million people who commit suicide could be much less and eventually be zero. The humiliation that those diagnosed with a mental illness feel will have disappeared, as the world is finally honest enough to admit that we are all equally vulnerable and it is for the benefit of the human race to always be open about our mental health and emotional problems. Madness will have been cured. The term mental illness will be redundant and Hubbard's and my mission will be complete.

A logical first step is to look at Hollywood liberalism itself. Let us analyse this in a simple form so that we all understand it. Think of the film As Good As it Gets starring Jack Nicholson. This is a film about a writer with Obsessive Compulsive Disorder but is never presented in this fashion in the public domain. It is advertised as being about a reclusive writer. The Obsessive Compulsive Disorder is the comic element. If the film were called "The Man with Obsessive Compulsive Disorder" instead, then would empathy for this condition in society be raised to a higher level? Would this lead to a greater increase in empathy of the real suffering of people, who endure this kind of condition in the public's consciousness? If so then why not promote As Good As It Gets as a film about Obsessive Compulsive Disorder?

1) Because it would not be appealing to the eye and it wouldn't sell? Possibly. People go to the cinema to be entertained and to switch off. They want to forget problems and go into a dream like state. Looking at recent films like Fahrenheit 9/11, serious documentary film makers have now proven that there is room for them to have a voice, and a real impact on the way that the world thinks.

2) Because comedy itself acts on a subliminal level and is often more serious than tragedy? Maybe. Just ask a comedian what drew them to

the profession, and analyse the mood swings of any comedian. There is a fine line between comedy and madness and they are often intertwined. A genius like Paul Merton (A comedian from England, for any American friends reading this) has been open about his manic depression since the early 90's. Think how many people he has helped just by announcing that. A lot. Think for a minute... if he starred in his own autobiography on manic depression in a Hollywood blockbuster... What a positive impact on mental health that would have. Also if Paul Merton can achieve this why can't I or you for that matter. Think how many people we could empower with mental health issues then.

3) Another reason why we don't promote 'As Good As it Gets' as a film about "Obsessive Compulsive Disorder" could be that there is no objective proof that this condition exists. It is a manufactured term like any other mental illness. The American Professor whose book I have published on behalf of Chipmunkapublishing, John Breeding, is exactly right when he says that "Philosophically madness is a social construct and psychiatry is a form of social control that is unrivalled since the Nazi's genocide of the Jews". Any intelligent Buddhist or spiritual healer should be able to articulate the value to one's health in understanding this line of thought. Although this is not yet a practical solution for us all, as people still find it difficult to create creative flows all of the time. However more and more people around the world understand this line of thought as the social evolution of curing

madness takes place. You have begun to understand as you have read this far. If only the owners of the world's pharmaceutical giants admitted this think how many people we could help.

4) The film As Good As it Gets is also not promoted as a film about OCD (we can now call it this for convenience) because world economics and drug companies are already doing this job for us. I'm not necessarily agreeing with this, just mentioning it as a possibility. The instant response here would be: "drugs help people like that so it is not our problem, and I do not want to be associated with somebody with Obsessive Compulsive Disorder anyway as that would cause stress in my life. Also if I get too close to it and understand it too well I may realise that I have it myself and so do people in my family. Then I will need medication and have to take pills for that on top of my Prozac. That would affect my drinking and nicotine patches".

5) Jack Nicholson is already the greatest madman on earth. How else would he be the most successful Hollywood actor of all time? (If you look at Oscar nominations he is). He is the man from One Flew Over the Cuckoo's Nest. There is no need to redefine him as a madman when the status quo has already been conditioned into unwittingly understanding his public persona. He has been deliberately typecast by the inner circle of Hollywood's major players to enlighten the world about what it is like to suffer

from madness as people still identify him with that film.

All five points raise the level of awareness of mental health. Now let's take it a step further. 'As Good As it Gets' is a powerful film that creates empathy for people with mental health problems and reduces stigma and discrimination against the mentally ill in the media and society. It helps to break down the taboo of mental health and stops people who need help being seen as axe wielding maniacs that go round killing others because they forgot to take their medication.

'A Beautiful Mind' has arguably done much the same thing. It shows so accurately the goings on and sufferings of the mind of a schizophrenic. The realisation when the audience sees that the star is actually mad is one of the most powerful moments in the history of cinema. It is the closest description to my own realisation and reflection of my manic rituals that I have ever seen, or even imagined, on the big screen and it is my goal to change the way Hollywood thinks and depicts the mental health of us all, so that must be a compliment (this drive within me is not to gratify my own ego or even to psychoanalyze myself but a humanitarian sensitivity to want to help other people).

Hollywood is such a powerful medium as it takes royal status in our consumerist culture. Film is such a powerful medium as it is everywhere, in and around us, what people model themselves on, idolise and daydream about being. It is on such a global scale. The moment in a great piece of cinema can live with us forever and change the way we think about something. This can of course be done directly and on a subliminal level. For Russell Crowe (who appeared in A Beautiful

Mind) perhaps it was even too much. I wonder was that why he punched that producer? Because he was so emotionally involved with that character that he did not want the words of his character edited. He had become like the *Freddie in The Nightmare On Elm Street* but for a good reason, to help people with mental illness. A Beautiful Mind broke new ground but could have gone even further if it had covered the major character's homosexuality or implied that the medication was part of the problem. Still there is only so much you can do with one movie.

As for the social evolution, visualise what is known by few as The Mental Health Movement i.e. people campaigning for equality for people with mental ill health – e.g. people with manic depression, schizophrenia, obsessive compulsive disorder, severe personality disorder etc... Compare the mental health movement to The Gay and Lesbian Movement for a moment.

In 1986 when I was eleven I noticed that Gay and Lesbian culture was not generally accepted. By the time I was nineteen in 1994 it was part of the social norm. In fact it was cool to be gay once people realised that HIV wasn't a gay disease. By 2054 it will be cool to have manic depression. Let's hope that by 2104 nobody will have a mental illness. I cannot express how urgent it is for us to work together on this. According to the World Health Organisation by 2020 suicide will be the second most common form of death. Figures are on the increase world wide so my predictions for 2104 need to be aimed for to stop a global epidemic. It makes drug companies money and is a form of social control so we're all bound to have something right?

The most natural way to get to this utopia for people who have experienced mental health issues is to fight for their civil liberties (as they have been doing quite noticeably since the 1960s, but not on a scale sufficient enough for the whole world to take any real notice) to be open about their own mental health issues.

As I was diagnosed with manic depression in 1993 I see both everything and nothing as a mental health issue. I have accepted what happened and overcome the humiliation, and as a result managed to cure myself. I realised that there was no mental health issue except the one created by society and my own mind and unconscious fears, insecurities and desires. I spend my life convincing others that everything is a mental health issue so that the taboo of mental health is broken down and that they realise that everything and nothing is a mental health issue at the same time. Once their unconscious fears have left, then the social evolution takes another step forward. That is what I am doing on a subliminal level. At a grassroots level I will always be open about my "condition" and encourage others to come out of the closet and be proud of who and what they are. Leaders are needed throughout the world to stand up and speak out.

Just because someone has manic depression or something similar doesn't mean that they should feel embarrassed. In fact experiencing madness, like any kind of struggle, gives an individual a greater capacity to bounce back and become a stronger person. Overcoming madness in particular gives you the potential power to help other people who go through the same experience. There is no greater feeling in the world than this, except for maybe true love, and having children. Once you help more and more people you begin to realise that you can in fact prevent the pain and suffering of others, you can avoid that negative state and feeling of isolation, humiliation, confusion and nothingness that being labelled and experiencing a mental illness brings.

Let's examine another two examples for the social evolution. Visualise Frank Bruno and Mike Tyson. Both former heavyweight champions of the world and both have been described as mad. Mike Tyson's madness has almost been an endearing part of his character. Mike's madness was part of his persona as the greatest knockout puncher in the most macho sport in the modern world. The madness in him (I remember fondly his cameo performance in the film Black and White where he quotes Nietzsche when giving some advice to his friend), his fighting, his training is part of the Tyson package. This is an example that madness is something that fascinates people, but not something that they want to get too close too. There are many people who admire Tyson and a few who say they would go in a ring with him, but a minute number when it actually boils down to it. Just imagine the fear of the madness when stepping in with Tyson when he was at his best. Like putting a psychiatric patient in a straight jacket, or having a meeting with your psychiatrist in a ward round for those of you who are more informed of the power imbalance in the psychiatric model. No chance and not therapeutic.

Now let's look at Bruno. He's a public hero. He was Britain's most loved man in many ways when I was growing up in the 1980s. In 2004 Frank Bruno was devastatingly taken into a psychiatric unit near to his home in Essex. The Sun had headlines of "Loony Bruno", as Britain's hero had become one of the institutionalised mentally ill. Marjorie Wallace MBE from SANE the most skilful PR mental health strategist of her generation from a mental health charity in the UK managed to have the tabloid change its headlines before the morning paper. What significance did this day bring. A very sad time for Frank Bruno, his friends and family of course, but this day will be looked back on again as a historic moment in 20 years time and onwards.

The day a public hero fell from grace and became one of the mentally ill. That was one of me, one of who I was. If it could happen to someone as loved as Frank Bruno then the rest of Britain would finally empathise and begin to understand what people with mental health issues go through. It would cease to be a taboo. It would be part of the social norm. Only a matter of time. For people would be forced to realise that their own mental health is perilously close to going over the edge.

Imagine this shift in consciousness doubling in size that day and doubling every subsequent month as the Bruno effect began to influence society. Then, improved communication amongst friends after work about their own mental health. Not embarrassed to talk about this anymore. Frank Bruno went through it; everyone likes Frank so I can talk about it and vice versa. Then this historical shift takes effect. If you believe in it, it will happen. Positive chi spreads.

Within fifty years a generation of people have began talking about their own mental health and it becomes as normal as watching a game of football in your home on SKY five years ago i.e. year after year it becomes more commonplace as people have gone before and it becomes more acceptable (in the case of mental health) and more affordable in the case of SKY SPORTS. Mental health becomes a commodity, a brand, like Virgin Records was the first and then 250 Virgin Companies followed to form the Virgin Brand. The same will happen with mental health.

My vision is that this will happen in the brand of Chipmunka. Why? Because everyday I take massive action[5] to do this, I am totally committed to it. Before I embark upon my vision further I would like to emphasize that the need to develop it does not come out of gratifying my own ego, fame or fortune but the understanding to follow on a humanitarian and anthropological impulse, an inevitable development in man/woman kind, where the world will demand a recognised Global Mental Health Brand. If it is called Virgin even better, it saves me a lot of work. My intention is not to repeat any other activities that are going on in the Mental Health Movements throughout the world but to have them plug in to each other so that they can all achieve maximum effect and work together to reduce suffering in the world. There is also nobody doing it the way that Chipmunka does it. We give people a voice as they tell their own story. It is not my role to care for people who have had mental illness. The mental health sector in the UK, and globally, has been doing excellent work in the past 40 years but based on the wrong premise. Generations of people with mental illness will never get better if they are

---

[5] The phrase 'massive action' is used by Anthony Robbins. For an introduction to motivational speaker Anthony Robbins read Unlimited Power, Published by Simon and Schuster 1989. Highly recommended.

cared for. They will only get better if they take control themselves. Anyone who understands the massive benefits of Neuro Linguistic Programming and newer more advanced techniques will understand that it comes from the individual. It is only the individual that can snap themselves out of a mental ill health mindset.

There is nobody doing it like Chipmunka. We produce products where people tell their own story. They have the voice. They are the leaders of their own destiny. Chipmunka is just the mechanism by which they do it. We are like their football agent. We positively discriminate in their favour.

On closer evidence it becomes apparent that the odds are stacked in Chipmunka's favour. It is impossible to usurp the pioneering body of something. The universe doesn't work like that. This can only be a good thing for society and people in general. With the raising of awareness of such a brand, more people get the help that they need. They do not feel as isolated as they were. They can rejoin society again.

CHAPTER ONE

CANS OF MADNESS

Episode 1: The Play

"I began writing a play of fiction when I was 19 years old about my first manic episode because I did not have the 'mental strength' to write this drama in the first person due to the humiliation that society made me feel and because of the way I self manifested my mental illness". The experiences of the character Will are largely based on my own experiences in real life. They illustrate my first steps to recovery in the sense that I managed to face up to my condition and also managed to sometimes laugh at my experiences. I also envisaged a happy ending which is a crucial part of the recovery process".

Will is a tall, confident, charismatic individual with a rather worn look about him. Smithers is his surname - walking round his apartment with big hand movements.

WILL: It's about time something went right. Could have been a millionaire by now or something, but no - stuck in that rut. Trapped in the world of man, the people aren't so bad; it's the governments, the media and religion that are to blame. The masses are nice enough, just boring, of course annoying, frustrating and aggravating, but so is life. Nothing everlasting except death. Only thing that's worth remembering is madness. A can of madness. It's in a class of its own. [Sets up a beer bong] A glass of its own, a jug, a jar, a crate, an offie, a wholesale, a world... [He necks the beer bong] There isn't any way out, at least there shouldn't be. That's the tragedy.

Flashback to 4 years previous at a rave with some friends; Will is rushing, looks at glen and cookie three times. Camera close up, firstly on Will and secondly on his mates. 30 seconds long accompanied to music.

NEIL: Coming up on those pills man. Absolutely off it. Me and Cookie are going to chill out "you'll be all right"-Yeh it's sorted here.
The club is hard-core like a cavern. A triangular dance floor with a balcony upstairs - everybody's fucked. Local DJs at the front are kicking it.

WILL'S HEAD: The music's getting louder. Will's coming up. Off it all right! He's the craziest fucker in there all right. He's so fucked he stomps all the way up the stairs round the whole fucking club.

WILL: all right mate

WILL'S HEAD: He shakes some fuckers hand whose been imitating him all night.

WILL: He's banging downstairs again. Can't even see. Will walks forward stomping from the back left to the middle right of the club. "Where's the MC?" [Louder] "Where's the MC?" [The dodgy looking sounds-man points towards the left. Will walks diagonally left and finds the MC].

WILL: [To some big fuck by the decks]. Say to Lomas that Johnny from 109 says hi.

BIG FUCK: What?

WILL: Say to Lomas that Johnny from 109 says hi.

BIG FUCK: Alright mate. [Hands Will a nice pill].

Will goes to the front of the club and stomps alarmingly robotically for five minutes. The club's night is over but not Will's, he's still fucked. Now this lads been e`d up before right, but he's always been highly charged you see. The Mc's Bacchanal like chant of hardcore becomes absorbed into Wills head.

WILL'S HEAD: Back At Will's mate's house everyone's off it, right. They're all chilled out, but this fuckers stomping 'til ten in the morning, then he's smoking spliff and necking vodka.

WILL'S HEAD: Next night's a Saturday and there's another party. This one's more pretentious, but still just as crazy. Fifteen hundred fuckers poncing about. Will's still stomping his head off, right.

The screen goes blank and a scream is heard. Aaaaaaaaahhhhhgg! The scream symbolises the plight of Will. Four hours later Will is woken up. He's taken into the bathroom by David, undressed and given a bath. Will does not speak he's confused and embarrassed. He is bathed by David, his head soaked with a flannel to clean the bruise. The water drains away and a towel is put round him, afterwards. Now Cookie and Glen are there and they're going with the flow, nothing too noticeable like, just chilling. Now, 20 hours stomping is enough to do anyone's head in, but not Will's. A five minute massage and he does not give a fuck. Only thing is two days later Will aint come down. In fact, two weeks later he's not come down but gone up, gone up so much he's in the bleeding local mental asylum for assaulting his brother. He's not sectioned right, but when the authorities ask him what he wants to do, he says he'll go.

They take him down the hospital for a brain scan and the daft twat thinks he's having his hair cut. He's taken down the cells 'cause they don't know what to do. After head butting the cell door for three hours continuously and left with a lump the size of a tennis ball on his head, they section him and take him down the bin. Yet this fucker, although he's in a straight jacket in the back of a police van, still thinks he's going off to a rave right. What are they gonna do with him? It's dark when he gets there and desolate. Only one night nurse there. Exhausted, Will goes to sleep. He's screaming 'cause his prick hurts. They've given him some drug, see.

NIGHT NURSE: It'll be o.k. Will. [She's holding his hand]. Come on Will, let's go to bed.

She takes him up to some dormitory and undresses him. Will curls up and goes to sleep.

Next morning at 8.00am this alarm sounds and within 30 seconds several Zombies are off to clean their teeth.

DAVID (MORNING NURSE): Nudging Will. Come on Will, wake up...Wake up.

LISA (A NURSE): [Calls to David from the corridor, but not in the room].Is he not coming up then?

DAVID: No. We'll leave him as it's his first day.

LISA: You sure?

DAVID: Yeh, there's no harm in that.

David cleans his teeth.

Four minutes later Will is in the lounge. The lounge is rectangular with seats for twenty people facing a large television. Separated by some bookshelves another half dozen seats are visible for those who want some more privacy. In the kitchen area, at the end of the hall is a table-tennis table. A gap in the wall where the food is dealt out and an old piano gives a physicality and nostalgia to the kitchen.

All is observed by the employees of the institution. They take it in turns to look out through the gap in their wall, one of the nurse's called Marge, is sat watching the TV with the others.

The following characters are shown interacting in the lounge:

A granny named Doris sits nearest the telly. She knits and chain-smokes. Adjacent is Phyllis, an identical old woman who is prone to knitting more and smoking less.

Graham is more of a loner at sixty years old. He's chain-smoking roll ups, has yellow and brown fingers and tends to bite his nails nervously. Graham is miserable, nostalgic and plays the piano. He has the tendency to talk incessantly to himself about old things such as the school he used to go to, the music he's heard and books he's read. When he's nervous he rests his head on his neck and bangs his knees up and down.

Stevie is fat, gay and over friendly; he sulks if nobody notices him. Stevie has a high pitched voice wears a pink cap back to front and wears luminous clothing. He looks more like a cartoon than a real person.

Terry moves a lot, to sit in different seats. Terry usually keeps quiet. He's a big bloke, an ex-skinhead, a tough nut who spends most of his time blagging cigarettes and looking at his knuckles. He gets into gardening eventually.

Lee attempted suicide. A volatile character, one minute he's laughing and the next minute he's devastated.

Nigel, on the same day his wife left him, he lost his job and admitted he was an alcoholic.

Marie is a fifty year old sophisticated lady. She's a part-time writer and is well spoken. Marie seems 'all together' but, is very depressed.

Martha is a 30 year old black chick with glasses. She has contradictory characteristics: pretty, friendly, talkative, nosey, stressed, neurotic and argumentative.

Simon is a university lecturer. He is in some sort of a relationship with Martha. He can be very arrogant and judgmental, but he is also very honest and an interesting personality. Simon wears glasses, is smartly dressed and has messy brown hair and crazy eyes.

Julian can be found with his legs bouncing nervously. He's either shouting 'Man. United' continuously or doesn't say anything for weeks.

Mark is a schizophrenic, he never speaks and is good at chess.

Martha, Simon, Stevie and Nigel all exit. Lee leaves the lounge, but then comes back. Winnie and Scott enter.

Will walks around in front of the television and calls each of them, in turn, a hardcore DJ.

WILL: You're Lomas, you're Carl Cox. Nice to meet you Stu Allen and you must be Top Buzz. I'm the MC, the muther fucking MC. Alrigghtt.

Will walks out of the lounge towards the nurse's room and meets David.

WILL: You're MC Tunes. I'm MC Will.

DAVID: Your mother and brother are here to see you.

WILL: HI MC Lennie! I'm MC Will. Come into the quiet room.

DOMINIC (Will's Brother): What's the quiet room? [Dominic has a broken nose].

WILL: It's just through here. [He signals to ten yards past the nurse's room]. Look at this lot. Isn't it great? Loads of it? Where's the DJ? Where's the DJ?

DAVID: If you make a mess Will, you're going to have to clear it up.

WILL: No, MC Lennie's gonna clear it all up. Ain't ya.

DAVID: [Talking to Dominic] He's pretty bad as you can see, but they all come in like this and they do get better. [Signalling to Will] Your brother's not going to clear it up Will. You'll have to, once you've finished.

WILL`S MUM: Is it drugs?

DAVID: We don't know yet. That's what it seems to be, but it's more complicated than that, it could be anything. Drugs are almost certainly part of it.

WILL: I'm the DJ, where's the MC? There you are!

DAVID: Stop it, that's enough now Will.

Will has thrown a stereo on the floor. Games, puzzles and all their pieces scatter over the ground.

WILL: You're going to clear it up [motioning to Dominic].

DAVID: No he's not. Why should he? You did it.

WILL: I know you're going to clear it up.

DAVID: Leave him tidying up and we'll have a chat.

WILL: This is the quiet room.

DOMINIC: [Smiling] I know...The quiet room.

The audiences' attention is drawn to shrieking in the background.

BACKGROUND VOICE: Get off o' me. Get off o' me right. You're dirty right. Get off o' me. Free me. Free me. Save me God. Get off o' me. Right, leave me alone. Who do you think you are? Give me a cigarette!

MARGE: What do you say?

WINNIE: Right.

MARGE: What's the magic word Winnie?

WINNIE: Please. [Takes the cigarette] Give me a fucking cigarette.

MARGE: That's not very nice, I gave you a cigarette and you say that. That's disgusting. Give me the cigarette back!

WINNIE: No... Ha, ha, ha. [She pulls a funny face].

MARGE: Did you see what Winnie did David?

DAVID: Yerh, that wasn't very nice, was it Winnie?

Will sits down, near where Graham usually is, and smokes a cigarette whilst hiding his packet.

MARGE: You can have the cigarette Winnie, I don't mind. It's dinner time in a minute anyway. Doris, will you help me serve out today's lunch?

Doris puts her knitting down and advances to the kitchen. Will observes this looking through the bookcase.

Will rushes to the canteen and is at the front of the queue. He is given a huge lunch and eats it all. By the time he reaches the pudding, he just sticks his mouth in it and eats the sponge cake with custard in one mouthful. His mother and brother look on with a look of horror, but are glad that he is, at least, eating.

At nine o'clock in the evening all Will's visitors have to leave. Thirty seconds of music here... Scene moves into the kitchen area.

DAVID: Would you like a game of table tennis then Will?

WILL: Give us a bat then.

DAVID: [There is dark lighting] When you beat me you can leave here.

Will gasps. He has now realised that he is living in a mental asylum. David wins quite easily, playing intelligently, cleverly and defensively. Will's not very co-ordinated at the moment.

It is now a few weeks later, Cookie is sat next to a cationic Will. There is quite surreal lighting. Will suddenly tries to speak but there is a pang in his jaw. He's crying from the pain. It is the worst moment of Cookie's life; his mate has turned into a cabbage, a fucking vegetable. Cookie's eyes are watering and he breaks down and cries on his way out.

Apart from his family, Cookie and Glen are Will's most frequent visitors. They seem to take it in turns visiting him and they brighten up Will's day. Glen helps a lot because he has just stopped pinging up billy. He knows what it's like being off your twat as he's still off his twat.

GLEN: Sorry I'm a bit late, I went down the gym.

WILL: It's alright

GLEN: I've put on twelve pounds in the last two weeks.

Will raises his eyebrows with sincere acknowledgement.

GLEN: I'm doing one hundred and fifty pounds on the bench press now.

Will raises his eyebrows once more, but this time a little higher.

WILL: How many repetitions?

GLEN: Ten. I'll be squatting eventually.

WILL: Yerh?

GLEN: I was thinking about me and Taylor earlier, on me way up 'ere. Them times in the squat were mad... Mad Will. I was staring out of a window right, and Taylor prodded me saying I'd been staring out that window for four hours. I thought I'd just been glancing at it.

WILL: You're madder than me. [Smiling]

GLEN: Remember that time round your house and your gran turned up. [Laughing] I'll never forget that. Cookie answered the door and ran up the stairs terrified of her 'e was. [Will smoke's a cigarette] We all 'ad them trips and that wiz. You 'ad to get to France the next mornin'.

I'll never forget the time you sparked out Graham Burgess. [Laughing louder] We all went round there on acid. You asked him to come out, so you could have a word with 'im, and decked 'im and started bootin his head in. He knew you woz gonna hit 'im but 'ey still came out.

36

WILL: Ey put his feet up in my kitchen. I had to hit him.

GLEN: What about that time when you knocked that copper over the 'ed. I couldn't stop laughing when you told us. Only you'd ran back in the van, you loon. Did you knock 'im out?

WILL: I pegged it and looked around thirty seconds later, he was crawling to someone's door to get 'elp. Worst thing was when Cookie threw away the CB I could have flogged that down the car boot sale. Well, at least I never got caught. I'd have ended up in borstal.

GLEN: What about when we did that shit bomb, with Jon's shit in that bag? I'd love to av seen the look on their faces when they saw it all over their patio windows.

You know, Fantasia was the best night of my life. What was it we 'ad? ....Doesn't matter, you know when I was down the squat I had a quarter in one ping. None of them down there 'ad as much as that, not even Johnny.

WILL: You're madder than me.

GLEN: Wanna game of table tennis, nutter?

WILL: Yeh.

They walk through the lounge of zombies into the kitchen area. Will's back is against the zombies and Glen is against the far wall. Will may look rather drug induced but his table tennis has improved whilst being locked in a vacancy. The ball shoots from side to side. Each shot looks a winner, but the other player is able to carry on. Rather like that scene in Terminator two when Arnold Schwarzenegger cripples the other Terminator with a shotgun, but the injured party is miraculously transformed and continues the chase with the utmost ease.

The score is 3-2 to Will and he serves like one of the Wongs in the Wanderers, throwing the ball three feet in the air and cutting it. Here the score appears on the screen to give the audience a sense of participation and continues until the game is finished.

Five all and Glen tries a smash, which lands in the middle of the lounge. Nearly in tears of laughter he retrieves the ball, 5-6 to Will.

Serving like Tommy out of 'Goodfellas' - return like Joe Pesci's death in 'Casino'.5-7. Serve like the policeman spitting on Larry Fishburne's mate in 'King Of New York' – response: he licks it up 5-8. Serve like a baseball swinger in the 'Warriors'. It's out 5-9. Serve like fat fucker loser in 'Full Metal Jacket' and returned like he ends up, a psychopath, 5-10. 11-5 classic Johnny Woo serve with perfect oriental direction. 11-6, Carling getting beaten up in 'Scum'. 12-6 smashed like Begbie in 'Trainspotting', unfortunately. 13-6, spin like agent Kuyon in the 'Usual Suspects'. 13-7, like Spartacus almost gets away with but doesn't quite. 7-14. Escape shot like Robert de Niro in the Russian roulette scene in 'Deer Hunter'. 7-15, as cool as Mr. Blonde in 'Reservoir Dogs'. 8-15, as helpless as John Travolta is when shot in 'Pulp Fiction'. 9-15, as sly as 'Dirty Rotten Scoundrels'. 9-16, as cool as Matt Dillon in the 'Flamingo Kid'. 16-10, missed serve. 16-11, four shots a piece, overpowered defensive shot. 16-12, the longest rally of the game and a fabulous winning smash. 17-12. Spin serve wins point. 17-13. Bad serve. 13-18. Bad serve. 14-18. Serve not returned hits the net. 14-19, fourth shot hits corner. 15-19, serve not returned. 16-19, serve not returned. 20-16. Eleventh shot smash. 20-17, bad serve. 21-17. Third shot of rally is a majestic back spin on the forehand which wins the game.

They both place their bats on the table. Glen sits in the lounge. Will grabs the ping pong balls, walks into the kitchen and puts them in the microwave where they soon explode.

GLEN: What did you do with them?

WILL: Put them in the microwave.

Glen laughs. Will proceeds to smoke a cigarette.

GLEN: I'll have to go in a minute; I've got a date tonight.

Will looks upset.

WILL: It's alright.

GLEN: I'll come tomorrow though, after I've been down the gym, same time. [Will offers Glen a cigarette]. No thanks Will I haven't smoked a cigarette for three and half weeks now... 'The Krays' is on tonight.

WILL: Yeh.

GLEN: Remember when we 'ad them mushrooms round your 'ouse. I couldn't count the money to get in the taxi and I had lunch with your old chap and Catherine. [Mad frown and laugh at the same time]. Them were the days. [Looking at his watch] Better be off then. See ya tomorrow mate.

They shake in mutual agreement of the next meeting. Will sees Glen out.

GLEN: See you tomorrow Will. [Raising his eyebrows]

Will is sitting in the rectangular quiet room. He is vigorously banging his feet up and down and chain smoking whilst listening to hardcore techno. Cookie walks in and acknowledges the frenzied repetitive beat immediately.

COOKIE: Alright Will. There's somebody to see you. [Lydney pops his head round the door]

LYDNEY: Alright Will. [Lydney is dressed like a DJ and behaves accordingly. His persona is flamboyant and jocular].

Will and Lydney join in male bonding, hugging of course, silly.

COOKIE: Oh by the way Will, I've got some stuff for you. Some chocolate and some pop.

WILL: I don't want that crap.

COOKIE: Well if you don't want me to bring anything then I won't.

LYDNEY: So how long you been crazy, Will? Noh, only joking. What you doing in here Will? You've gotta get out of this place. Everybody's crazy in here. This bloke on the way in right, he looked like a ghost. No seriously man, I thought he was a ghost. In fact, I still think he is a ghost.

Lydney still offers Will a cigarette. Will takes one although he has a plentiful supply.

Man you've got your own cigarettes. Still... doesn't matter this once, does it? As long as it's just once. Still at least you're not as bad off as Steve. You're not going to believe what he did Will. Check this out man. This is the funniest thing you're ever going to hear. Man, your not going to believe this. [Cookie laughs]. Poor Steve... He's in his room right. Oh by the way nobody else knows this right. Well nobody's supposed to know. But it's so funny man. It's soooooo funny, I have to tell it. Listen to this right, Will. Steevo is in is room right, you know he can't pull any birds right. Well he's got hold of this battery operated vibrator right, from his sister's room. It was a present from her boyfriend for her birthday. Anyway, he's got hold of this vibrator right and he's fiddling around with it.

He puts some cream on it. The next bit's disgusting man, don't say I didn't warn you. He sticks it up his arse hole and switches it on full speed. Now this cream was the wrong sort of cream, coz he electrocutes himself. Some time later his sister opens his door probably wondering where her toy has gone, as her boyfriend is working late and her brother's lying there unconscious with her precious vibrator up his arse. He had to go to the hospital and stay there overnight for his drunken antics and ribald buffoonery. Now if I go round there, his sister won't speak to 'im. She hasn't spoken to him since, poor cow. Now what do you think of that?

Will seems to have been listening tentatively but is rather sedated and frowns whilst reaching for one of his own cigarettes.

I thought that would 'av cheered you up? It certainly cheered me up.

COOKIE: Anyone else been to see you today Will?

WILL: Yeh, Glen.

LYDNEY: I haven't seen Glen for ages. How is old Glen?

COOKIE: ...He's alright. He's stopped injecting now. He goes down the gym most nights.

LYDNEY: I remember old Glen. Everything that kid did, he always did it to excess. He was dead against drugs for ages, wasn't he? Then he ended up being the one who pinged up. Yep, he's a nutter. He's always been a nutter. Remember when he came round when we had those strawberries? He had a funny look on 'im then, as though he didn't approve or something.

COOKIE: He soon made up for it though didn't he.

LYDNEY: Anyone up for a game of table tennis. I'm gonna whip ya Will.

They proceed into the lounge and Will goes into the kitchen to get a glass of water for Lydney. Cookie has the pop. Cookie and Lydney are playing when Will goes back into the kitchen. He makes a cup of tea with milk in it.

One of Nigel's visitors is just coming out of the kitchen and says hello to Will. Will gives a somewhat muted acknowledgement. Suddenly, Will pours the cup of tea over this middle-aged man's head. The man curses loudly and David rushes in. He looks physically threatening and asks Will to give an explanation for his behaviour.

NIGEL`S VISITOR: It doesn't matter; it wasn't boiling, just warm.

DAVID: But that's not on.

NIGEL`S VISITOR: It doesn't matter, leave it. He's only a young lad for Christ's sake. Look at him.

Cookie and Lydney look on intensely. Cookie puts his hands in front of his eyes in disbelief whilst Lydney shakes his head. That's the last time Lydney's going to visit.

DAVID: Lads I think you'd better go; it's almost nine o'clock anyway.

Lydney and Cookie look at Will. Will stares through them.

LYDNEY: Alright if we go now Will?

COOKIE: I'll come back and see you tomorrow Will.

WILL: [Shakes hands with Cookie]. Yeh, thanks for coming.

The next morning Will is sat down in the lounge smoking a cigarette bored, depressed, lonesome, frustrated, irritated and spaced out. His father walks in.

WILL`S DAD: Hiya, Will.

Will picks up the chair opposite him and runs with it, hurling it through the window.

WILL: Aaaaaahhhhhhhgggghhhh.

Will's Dad goes bright red and begins to cry whilst Will glares at him. Sat in the room between the quiet room and the lounge Will is chatting to an old woman who looks uncannily healthy. It's his grandmother. She hands him two different packets of cigarettes which he grabs eagerly.

WILL: Everyone's doing my head in.

OLD WOMAN: What do you mean 'doing your head in'? Do I do your head in?

WILL: Yeh. You do my head in... Everyone does my head in.

The old woman looks hurt and her lips start to quiver accordingly.

OLD WOMAN: You've never told me that I do your head in. Do I always do your head in?

43

WILL: Not always. It's this place that does my head in.

OLD WOMAN: I know it does but, I don't do your head in, do I?

WILL: Everybody does my head in. Not just you. My head's done in. Look at it. I'm doing my head in.

OLD WOMAN: I'd better go now.

WILL: O.K. Thanks for the cigarettes.

OLD WOMAN: It's O.K.

The woman leaves rather abruptly and is obviously very upset. Will seems rather annoyed as he did not mean to upset her, but he is glad that he has some more cigarettes to pass away his repression and boredom.

Will is alone in the quiet room dancing his head off to some hardcore- the rave that never was, but should have been. Glen walks in, glad that Will's off his head having a laugh. He mimics a hardcore night of a rush coming on, whilst heading for the tape deck.

GLEN: Wicked tune. Alright Will. Check this tape out you've gotta hear it. It's mental.

WILL: Yeh?

GLEN: Listen to this... Ever dreamt about a nuclear war?

Glen is smiling and nodding his head in little movements. The music starts, it's mad transcendental brain altering techno...Glen gradually turns up the volume and gives quicker and more violent nods of his head. Glen lights a cigarette sits down and starts dancing with it. Will continues being mental.

WILL: Nuff man dead fiddi I know.

GLEN: Come with us and go with the flow.

Glen turns the sound down and Will, still happy but not ecstatic, sits down and takes one of the cigarettes that Glen is offering.

GLEN: What d'ya think then? [Will smiles]. It's my maddest tape at the moment. I play it every night. You can 'av this I've made a copy for ya.

WILL: Thanks Glen.

GLEN: It's alright mate. How are ya then?

WILL: Bored until you cum.

GLEN: You're looking betta… Not so spaced out. Alright if I 'av a glass of water?

WILL: Water?

GLEN: Yeh, I'm thirsty from today's gym session [Stretching]. Pretty knackered actually.

Glen's looking at Will, who gets up and walks through the room of his bin colleagues. He retrieves two plastic beakers, as they are pretty small glasses, and fills them up with water. Will drinks one of them and fills it up again and walks past his fellow bin acquaintances, glancing at them watching the telly intensely.

Terry asks if Will has any cigarettes. Will shakes his head. He's thinking 'my fucking hands are occupied anyway you stupid cunt. How could I even give you a cigarette without spilling the two glasses of water'? Of course, Terry is rather self obsessed and doesn't give a fuck about anyone else. Something that is inevitable when you are crazy, you enter a world of your own and find it more interesting than the world which you have apparently left.

Will gives Glen the glasses of water.

GLEN: Cheers mate, there's two glasses?

WILL: You said you were thirsty.

Will leaves the room and ventures into the bathroom. He marches into each cubicle removing the toilet rolls from the holders and drops them into the toilets. Will then goes to the toilet feeling satisfied that he has completed his mindless daily ritual.

Will leaves the toilet, walks past the room Glen is in and advances towards his bedroom, which is on the ground floor as he has been rather disturbed lately. It is the only bedroom on the ward and kept for the, seemingly, most ill patient so they don't bother themselves or any of the other patients on the ward.

Sick of this military regime, Will has an idea. He goes back into the quiet room and opens the curtains, which lets the sun in. Will places a rucksack on his left shoulder filled with clothes and carries a handful of clothes in the other hand.

GLEN: What are you doing? [Laughing and still recovering from pinging up, Glen watches Will put on several pairs of socks, jeans and jumpers].

WILL: I'm going.

GLEN: [Hysterically] Where you going?

WILL: I don't know, but I'm going somewhere.

Glen erupts with laughter and can't stop. Will has put on all the clothes that he possibly can, puts the rest in the rucksack and walks around the room looking like he's been on steroids for five years.

GLEN: Do you know where you're going yet?

WILL: Out of here. [Will walks out of the quiet room and into the staff room]

I'm getting out of here. [Will walks into the lounge]

I'm getting out of here. [Will walks back into the quiet room]

WILL: I told you I was getting out of here.

Glen explodes with laughter once more and Will sits down.

Will is sat on a bench inside the hospitals grounds. Birds are singing and Will is accompanied by his brother Dominic and the old woman, his grandmother.

OLD WOMAN: Do you want a sandwich?

WILL: I'm sick of it 'ere.

DOMINIC: Would you like a sandwich?

OLD WOMAN: Oh shut up Dominic. Can't you see he's upset? [Dominic raises his eyebrows vehemently]. What's wrong darling?

WILL: I'm just sick of it.

OLD WOMAN: I know it won't be long now. This horrible nightmare's nearly over.

Dominic accordingly relaxes his eyebrows.

WILL: I'm so bored.

OLD WOMAN: Can't you read or something?

WILL: I can't concentrate for more than five minutes.

OLD WOMAN: Isn't there something you can do? Some sort of hobby or exercise to keep you engaged?

WILL: There is circuit training in the mornings but it starts at 8.00am.

OLD WOMAN: It might do you well to get up in the morning.

DOMINIC: Mornings? Yes. There's nothing wrong with getting up early in the mornings, you know you can see the hills, the sky and the postman if you get up early enough.

OLD WOMAN: Yes it might be just the thing you need, to get up early in the morning, get you back into some routine. Take it from me if you've got no routine then you've got nothing to get up for and nothing to do. If there's nothing for you to do then you're, more often than not, going to be bored or depressed.

WILL: Maybe.

OLD WOMAN: It's not a maybe, take it from me. Do what I say Will and believe me, you will feel better. If not, then at least you've given it a try and at least you've tried something different.

DOMINIC: You've put a bit of weight on as well you know bro.

Slapping Will in the chest, his brother smiles and Will's attempt at smiling is also partly successful.

OLD WOMAN: You could cut down on your cigarettes as well you know? But that's for you to decide. There's no hurry. I smoked for over sixty years and I still gave up you know.

Will, we had better get off. Dominic has got to sign on and I've got to get some vegetables from the market. You'll look back on this whole experience one day and realise that it's strengthened you mentally. You will, I promise. Believe me. You wait and see. Goodbye darling, we shall come and see you tomorrow. [She kisses him, Dominic and Will shake hands]. Take it easy. [Smiling, but more as a forced grin]

WILL: See you later bro.

DOMINIC: Later bro.

Next morning sure enough Will is off to do some exercise. It's about time really; he's been a miserable, lazy and headshot bastard for quite a while now. It's not necessarily his fault, but he's at last bucked up his ideas and decided to do something positive. It doesn't matter how trivial a thing he is doing, but it's important that he's made a decision to do something.

He has a brief conversation with Marge about him being up so early. The simpleton is only trying to do her job but reminds Will how many of the simpleton's ramblings he is forced to deal with everyday.

The song 'Football's coming home' is in the background and commentary is heard with the ensuing game.

Will arrives at the gym first. Soon, a couple of other zombies are queuing up outside the same door, when what looks like two junior school teachers appear. They both, a man and a woman, greet everyone with bland, vagrant and condescending 'hellos'. Will wants to puke. Will was once the school rugby captain of his grammar school and top goal scorer in his previous football career. He is, therefore, dumbfounded at the thought of a ten pounds overweight slob, bouncing a plastic football, believing he can teach Will anything about anything. Even worse for Will, the obese instructor proceeds to introduce himself, but reminds Will that he is a newcomer. He then adds that he hopes Will would choose to continue to go to his fitness classes.

The door is un-padlocked and opened. The zombies start kicking the football around as the two trainers attempt to gather them round in a circle. The effort is successful, but only as successful as it would be for a gym teacher to control a bunch of eleven year olds, with his militaristic tactics and accompanying whistle.

The exercises are for retards. Standing up, with one's feet apart, one bends over and tries to touch the ground keeping one's legs straight and one's fingers stretched. This is repeated three times at the front then back to the starting position; three times in the middle and three times underneath one's thighs. Everybody then proceeds to roll their shoulders vigorously forwards, then a break and the reverse procedure. The next loosener is to roll one's head round and round.

Having missed out other stretches some may deem important, the overweight instructor picks teams. Will, somewhat bewildered, stretches his ankles by rolling them either side and loosens his calves by putting one foot in front of the other and bending the front leg forward. Then intentionally catching the woman instructor's eye he stretches his back by putting his hands behind his back and pushing his hands up.

There are three people on Will's team and four on the other. The woman instructor leaves. She has only come to open the gym and gloat on and be offended by, psychotic penises, which can't even threaten the frigid bitch, as their beholders are mentally deranged for the foreseeable future.

The game starts as most football games start. A simple tap and the receiver tries to run past the opposing team and score on his own. In a fluke, passing one man, the attacker is floored by a good crunching tackle by Will's team mate. He then coolly passes back to the keeper who is rather slow but just manages to get the ball to Will. Will goes past two men and thumps the ball wide. Confronted by Fat-trainer-ma', who thinks he put Will off, Will is told he was unlucky.

WILL`S HEAD: How am I supposed to score with that fucking shite ball anyway? It's fucked. Just like me and this lot, all of them. I might as well kick a boulder of the same size. I got more chance of scoring with that. I could get more power behind it!

The other team scores a flukey goal. One of those goals that have a lucky ricochet and the scorer actually thinks he's a good player. Not even for one moment can he admit of his spawn.

Fat-trainer-man gives a smug grin and Will, in his trance like state, feels like a supplicant. Spurred on by going a goal down, Will's team give new meaning to what should be a John Wayne saying: 'Something good usually comes out of something bad'. They equalise immediately with what actually looked like and was, a good team goal. Two passes, a one two and a tackle maniac zombie-man side foots it past the goalkeeper.

At the restart, the opposition start how the rest of football matches start. Two passes and back to the goalkeeper. A feckless kick. Will intercepts, his shot rebounds off the goalie and trainer-man puts the ball into an empty net.

WILL`S HEAD: The goalie had come out, you see, that's the thing when it's rush goalie, you get knackered and get caught if you lose possession.

Fifteen more minutes and Will's team lose 4-3, but with three men that's not bad. The ball's so shite that nobody could score, especially Will. He had plenty of opportunities, but just could not score.

FOOTBALL COMMENTATOR: They've finished for the day and they're sweating like rapists. In fact, they would be rapists if they had the guts and could get away with it. Bet that's what it is to some of the women bin members, that's why they broke down. That's why they broke up. Up or down, does it really matter, there's still no way out.

Next time we see Will, he's in the lounge with two new faces. Lee and Neil are two older friends both none the wiser. They're both able to take a cynical, satirical and constantly hysterical view to Will's clinical insanity.

NEIL: You're not mad. At least you're conscious of what's happening.

LEE: You're crazy. [Laughing] You're crazy and you always have been. Crazy... Fucking Crazy.

Both of them laugh incessantly. Will's happy to see both of them but frowns, speechless with his mouth open.

NEIL: No, seriously you'll be alright. You're no crazier than me nor Lee, you're just the one it happened to, that's all. Don't worry about it.

LEE: Yerh, don't worry about it you cocksucker. I know people who're crazier than you.

NEIL: Yerh, your brother.

LEE: Dominic.

NEIL: Now he's really fucked.

Both continue laughing incessantly, just like a double comedy act. Except, they're not aiming to be funny, they're sad, predictable, selfish psychopaths.

Nevertheless, they brighten up Will's day and always have done. There's a real intensity with them, not like with Cookie and Glen. That's more relaxed. Here there's no such thing as respect. The rules are, there ain't no rules.

Amidst the riotous laughter Will's mother walks in with a muted and concerned smile.

WILL: Hi mum.

NEIL: Don't worry, we're not corrupting him or feeding him any drugs or anything. Not that these people don't seem to think so that is. I guess you've heard that they thought I was giving him drugs? As if. My Dad came up and had a right go at them. Anyway how are you?

WILL'S MUM: Alright thank you Neil. How are you Lee?

LEE: Oh, I'm alright.

WILL'S MUM: Don't worry, I won't tell anyone that you were here. Not anyone in particular.

LEE: [Sarcastically] thank you.

NEIL: Is the person in question Mr. Smithers, by any chance here? Does he still wish to… how can I put it? Want to have a quick word with you Lee?

LEE: I think he wants more than a quick word, more like a brawl or something.

Will's mother nods her head.

NEIL: Well, it's not surprising that after Will sang songs all day about Lee being a drugs dealer, that he wants to give you a jolly good old boot, old boy. What have you got to say to that Will? Eh?

WILL: I was only telling the truth. Anyway I can't really remember it.

Will runs out of cigarettes and looks rather startled as a result.

NEIL: Well, we'd better be off anyway. We're playing tennis this afternoon. Bet I'll win. Still you've got to play against someone, haven't you? Hurry back to normal Will and we'll have a game, you can borrow my racket... See you later and don't worry about it. You're alright, just the same as us really... Goodbye to Will's Mum.

WILL: See ya Neil. See ya Lee.

WILL`S MUM: Shall we get some cigarettes from the shop?

WILLL: Which shop? The shop inside the hospital?

As Neil and Lee exit, Lee distracted by one of the inmates, proceeds to miss the open door and walk into the wall, bashing his head.

LEE: You see what you've done to me Will? I'll be in here next and not just coming to see you.

Lee starts a mad cackle which is rhythmically accompanied by Neil. The two howling wolves leave.

Will's MOTHER: You o.k.?

WILL: Yeh.

MUM: Lee didn't do your head in?

WILL: No.

MUM: Good.

WILL: It was good to see them.

MUM: I`m sure it was.

WILL: You alright?

MUM: Yes dear, why shouldn't I be?

WILL: Just asking.

MUM: Don't be silly

WILL: I`m not. [Smiling]

MUM: They'll keep you in for longer if you're silly.

[Will groans vigorously but quietly]

MUM: Are we going to the shop then? [Grabbing her handbag]

She begins to rise and Will is slow, but uniform, in his effort to stand up. Some pensive music begins as Will is sulking, looking at the floor.

MUM: Coming then? What are we going to get?

They walk outside of the lounge and through the door. There is only a left turning and they walk down a corridor, which has a painting on the right hand side of the wall. The painting on the wallpaper covers the length of the whole corridor. Green trees, birds and blue sky represent an idyllic landscape yet look grossly out of place in such a madhouse. Will walks down the corridor with his palms brushing the painting. His mother looks round and asks:

MUM: What are you doing?

WILL: Painting.

A kind, but forced smile reaches her face as the doors of the corridor confront her. A forceful nudge opens the door, but only just. The next corridor is brighter and seems twice as wide. Yet the corridor's lighting is in the wrong place and it is actually dark. The seeming brightness is only for a nanosecond. The corridor has no windows. Twenty yards on the right hand side is a door but the camera is drawn to somebody who is twenty yards away from the end of the corridor, when Will and his mum walk in. The camera zooms in and concentrates on this overweight bloke in jeans and trainers smoking a cigarette. Then a sound is heard in the background which is the shop door opening.

The shop is three metres wide and three metres long. Will has less than three metres on the shop floor. The cashier in the shop is a sweet looking girl whom Will thinks is beautiful and mistakes for some E headed tart. Will grabs some Lucozade and proceeds to smother it in his left arm. Then he gets a Bounty bar, a Mars bar, two cans of Sprite and four packets of crisps.

WILL`S MUM: How about some cigarettes as well?

Will knows what cigarettes he wants, low tar Silk Cut, but his attention is drawn to the girl behind the counter. He cannot contemplate the room, which reeks of civilisation yet, is in bin surroundings. It was even more alien without the lemon and lime colouring of the rooms. Irritably alien, as Will is constantly reminded of societies conventions. If he would have been left in his own enlightening madness then he would have no worries or misgivings, in fact, he would be deliriously happy. Eventually he speaks.

WILL: Twenty Marlborough Lights.

WILL'S MUM: Make it forty.

Will look's at his mother in sombre thankful tone. The girl reaches over her right hand side for two packs of Marlborough Lights and she puts them on the desk.

WILL: Thanks but make it one pack.

MUM: Good. Are you going to those fitness classes again tomorrow? Do you want to go for a coffee now?

GIRL: That's on the house. Don't tell anyone.

Before hearing the price of the items, a crescendo of mind blowing techno is heard, the producer at Universe. The camera zooms in on Will's right wrist, which is violently shaking. The camera subsequently zooms into his head and then inside of his brain. (Bad Taste style)

Will is having a flashback. Surreal camera work is needed for this scene, therefore, no sense of time. Lydney and Glen are in a room. The curtains are open and flowers are in the background amidst a sloping driveway. The lounge is rectangular. There are two sofa chairs on the left hand side and a settee on the opposite corner. A television forms a right angled triangle. The sun shines through the window.

LYDNEY: Man, nothing happens, we've been conned just face it.

WILL: What time was it?

LYDNEY: We've been waiting for nearly two hours now. It's only supposed to take an hour.

WILL AND LYDNEY: Did you see that?

WILL: What?

LYDNEY: What d`you see man? What d`you see man?

WILL: The wall's breathing.

LYDNEY: Seriously.

WILL: Yerh.

LYDNEY: Noooo way. Nooo way. I saw the same thing, that's amazing really amazing. We've been sat here for two hours and seen nothing. Then suddenly bang. [Lydney gives a mad cackle] Wow they're moving.

Lydney is sat on the left hand side on the floor. Will is sat to his right, behind Lydney. Will motions to respond to Lydney`s remarks but then gulps, refrains from conversation and has suddenly fully realised that he's on his first trip and it has nowhere nearly ended yet. All the colours in the room have become more colourful since they came up.

LYDNEY: Woooow! The curtains are moving. See those patterns on the curtains. Look!

WILL: Lydney? [somewhat pensively]

LYDNEY: Not now Will, their zigzagging. Oh my god. This is great. Ha, ha, ha, ha. I don't believe it.

In the background a ringing is heard. It's the phone.

LYDNEY: Is that the phone? Nooo, is it? I've got to go and see if that's the phone. Wooohoo. Oh my god, that is the phone. Go on, pick it up. See who it is. Go on.

Will picks up the phone and suddenly looks dumbfounded. Glen is on the other end of the phone.

GLEN: Alright Will? Will rapidly hands the phone over to Lydney.

WILL: Speak to him. I can't speak to him; he'll do my head in.

LYDNEY: No way, you speak to him. I'm not speaking to him. I'm having a great time. I'm not gonna spoil it. I'm going back in the lounge. You can speak to him.

GLEN: Will is anyone there? Will?

WILL: ...Strawberries man

GLEN: Strawberries is that what you said? ....What do you mean strawberries?

WILL: Nothing Glen.

GLEN: You said strawberries.

WILL: No reason, I just said it.

GLEN: Yeh right.

WILL: No seriously. We've just had some Spliff.

GLEN: Yeh? [Interrogatively]

WILL: Yeh, were fucked. Come round if you want.

GLEN: Well, I dunno. I might do. I might see you later I might not.

WILL: Yeh.

GLEN: I might see you later, I might not.

WILL: Yeh.

GLEN: I might see you later then.

WILL: Yeh. Bye.

The conversation ends. By now Will is paranoid as hell. Lydney is not a sympathetic ear. Lydney advances towards Will and stops in front of him.

LYDNEY: I can't believe you told him we were on acid. He doesn't like drugs much, old Glen, does he Will?

WILL: I never told him we were on acid

LYDNEY: He knows though it's obvious.

WILL: Do you think he'll come round?

LYDNEY: Of course he'll come round, he's nosey.

Will is even more distraught and rings up Gavin.

WILL: Gavin. Listen right I`m on acid and it's doing my head in right. I've just spoken to Glen and I've told him we're stoned, but I don't think he's bought it. Come round if you want, but stop him coming round here. Please.

GAVIN: Alright. I'll see what I can do. [Laughing] Who are you there with?

WILL: Don't bring him round Gavin, please.

GAVIN: Alright. [Laughing] I'll see what I can do.

WILL: Are you coming round then?

GAVIN: Yeh, I'll see you in a bit.

WILL: You sure?

GAVIN: Yeh. [Laughing] See ya in a bit.

Lydney shouts from the lounge.

LYDNEY: Come and look at these curtains Will, they got mad patterns on them, look.

Will floats into the lounge almost.

Woow Ha ha ha ha ha ha hab ha. Wonder if I can get traces yet. Do you know what, I reckon I can. [Lydney moves his hands up from the armchair and waves them rapidly] Woow aaaaahhhhh. Wooow haaaaahaahaa. This is unbelievable, unbelievable! Watch it, hi-ya... hi-ya.... hwooah hwooooah. I love acid. I`m gonna take tonnes of it. My mates are all lightweights not to have taken more.

The doorbell rings and Will glides towards the front door opening it. Gavin and Glen are stood there. Gavin gives a cheesy grin whilst Glen looks aggravated.

Then Will is back in the bin, a euphemism for mental asylum of course, having a coffee and do-nought in the canteen. Will feels absurdly normal. He didn't know this place existed. His mother's theme of conversation tries to analyse how happy she is that Will is getting better. Unfortunately for Will, narking inside of his mind is the exact moment when he first entered this room.

WILL`S HEAD: One night in the bin the Krays had just finished and Will was sat with Terry. They all heard a thud, at least I think they all did.

JULIAN: Why don't you go and investigate Will?

Will look's for Terry's approval, who nods his head.

TERRY: Yeh go on Will.

Will walks out into the corridor. The painting can just be seen along the wall. He opens the door and comes to a right hand turning. Five yards on there is a closed green door. Will looks under the door and can see an empty room that looks like a large dentist's surgery. With increased ringing in Will's ears he focuses on the bed in the middle of the room. A metal bed without a blanket, Will can see two metal zigzagged strips hanging from the ceiling, or so it appears anyhow.

Will takes some tapes from out of his pocket and throws them down a metal drain which is right next to him. He breaks them in half. Before doing so he looks under the door imagining somebody bolted to the bed. He goes into a controlled frenzy, pulling his hair he gets up from the floor and heads further down the corridor. At the end of the next corridor on the right hand side is another door. This time it's red. He walks into the same canteen that he's eating his do-nought in. Straight ahead is where you get served. Towards the left are chairs. Will proceeds to piss on the coffee machine. He then picks up a broom and smashes the fuck out of the canteen. He only needs to hit things once, as they either smash to pieces or fall to the ground. Just starting to relax he puts a can in the microwave. By the time it has blown up he is sat on the canteen desk top, smoking a cigarette, completely calm and at peace. Night nurse two enters.

NIGHT NURSE 2: What the bloody hell you doin?

He pushes Will, and then continues to nudge him out of the room. Will concedes and the screen switches back to Will sitting back in the canteen, smoking a cigarette the do-nought and coffee finished. His mother's cup is nearly full. She's just finished a sentence.

WILL'S MUM: Out soon you know?

WILL: What?

WILL'S MUM: They're thinking of letting you out soon, you know? But they don't want you to get ill again, like last time. You're seeing Dr. Bailey again tomorrow.

In the doctor's office, which happens is also the quiet room.

DR.BAILEY: Hello Will. How are you?

WILL: Bored.

DR.BAILEY: I know it must be frustrating for you. How do you feel in yourself?

WILL: Bored, lonely, tired, drugged up, smothered, excited and claustrophobic.

DR.BAILEY: Excited what makes you feel excited?

WILL: The thought of getting out.

DR.BAILEY: And that makes you feel excited, does it?

WILL: Well, nervous actually.

DR.BAILEY: Nervous?

WILL: Yes.

DR.BAILEY: What are you nervous of exactly?

WILL: People laughing at me.

DR.BAILEY: What makes you think people will laugh at you?

WILL: Because, I've been in here.

DR.BAILEY: What if they don't know that you've been in here?

WILL: Then I can still feel them laughing, almost.

DR.BAILEY: Why?

WILL: Because, I know I've been in here

DR.BAILEY: Well that's what I'm here for. To help you come to terms with what has happened to you and to help you, to help yourself to feel better, if I can.

WILL: Feel better?

DR.BAILEY: Well, yes. I'm here to make you feel better and if you want me for anything else than I'll try and help you with that as well. Or if you want me just to talk with you, then I'm here for that as well and only that if you wish.

WILL: I don't mind talking to you.

DR.BAILEY: Well, thank you and why is that, do you think?

WILL: Because, I can say something daft and you laugh.

DR.BAILEY: Well, thank you, I think? I'd like to hope that I only laugh when it's funny, that I get the joke, O.K? Oh by the way, I forgot to say, I have to go a bit earlier today. I'll still have time to speak to Dr. Godray though. Anyway, we still have some time to talk. What would you like to talk about? Is there anything in particular?

WILL: Yes.

DR.BAILEY: And what would that be?

WILL: What do you think? They'll let me go?

DR.BAILEY: You mean let you go back home? Well, that's what I shall speak to Dr. Godray about this afternoon. Hopefully, if you keep progressing and getting better, next time we see each other it will be you coming to see me, not the other way round.

WILL: Would that be next week?

DR.BAILEY: Yes, if that's o.k. with you and it's o.k. with Dr. Godray then that's what we can all work towards very soon.

WILL: Yes.

DR.BAILEY: It's O.K. with you?

WILL: Yerh.

DR.BAILEY: Good then, fingers crossed. Is there anything else that you would like to talk about?

WILL: No.

DR. BAILEY: Well I'm sure you've been through the worst of it now. In fact you seem perfectly fine to me. What has been a bad dream can now be an awakening, if you choose to call it that. If you don't then it's no problem whatsoever. Oh, is that the time already? I'll go and speak to Dr. Godray now then and see what he says. You wait here if you like? That's it, have a cigarette, I shan't be long. If you're not in here when I get back I'm sure I'll find you.

Will lights a cigarette and walks into the staff room with it.

DAVID: You're not allowed in here Will, especially not with a cigarette. Will stays still. But... as you're going soon we'll let you off for a change. Dr. Bailey chatting to Dr. Godray now is he? Shall we have that game of table tennis then?

Will's eyes roll from right to left. They walk into the communal hall and start playing table tennis.

DAVID: Which side do you want Will mate?

Will shakes his head.

DAVID: Alright if I choose then? Will nods in agreement.

They start playing. In the first rally, David hits the ball into the lounge; Will runs into the centre of the room and picks up the ping pong ball. They play whilst Will smokes his cigarette and start scoring when he puts it out. Will wins the game quite comfortably. With six months practice this is not a great surprise.

DAVID: Looks like you've done it. Advancing towards Will and shaking his hand. Well done mate. Hardcore uproar right?

Will smiles nervously.

DAVID: Let's go in the staff room and have a cup of tea Will.

They walk towards the staff room. Will glances at the telly on the way and looks at the routine way in which everybody is sat glued to it.

TERRY: Have you got a cigarette Will?

Terry takes the cigarette and puts it on his ear. Will stands observing him whilst David goes back into the staff room to make coffee. Terry has tattoos on his fingers and one of an Asp on his arm. He sits down bouncing his legs up and down, then frowns, and holds his unlit cigarette at both ends. He stares at the cigarette turning it round with his left hand, and then puts it back onto his ear. Will then walks off. His back is turned when Terry calls him. Will turns round and Terry says Thanks.
Will now walks into the staff room and sits down. Lisa is in the staff room as well.

LISA: David's just told me that you're going soon Will. What d'you think about that then? Pleased I bet? Fed up of us old fogies in here then?

DAVID: Here's your coffee. I should think you'll be glad to see yourself out of here Will. We're all sick of the sight of you anyway. No... only joking!

WILL: Hardcore uproar.

LISA: What's that mean? Hardcore uproar?

DAVID: It's Will's invention, it just took him a while to wait for it to happen that's all.

LISA: Oh I see now

WILL: Hardcore uproar.

Dr. Godray and Dr. Bailey enter the little room. Dr. Godray is a tall man with a blue suit. He's very sensible looking. Dr. Godray smiles at everyone, nods his head at David and winks at Will.

DR. GODRAY: Bye and see you next week Will...oh, and by the way, that's at my office not yours.

Will gives a tentative sigh of relief.

DAVID: Shall we go into the interview room then Will, for our last chat.

They walk in the small room and sit down.

DAVID: So you're out in a few days?

WILL: Yep.

DAVID: What are you going to do with yourself then, as soon as you get out?

WILL: Go to McDonalds.

DAVID: And have a Big Mac meal?

WILL: Yep, with super size fries.

DAVID: What are you going to do with your life?

WILL: Nothing. Just study.

DAVID: What are you going to do to yourself?

WILL: Nothing. Get drunk

DAVID: You gonna take drugs again?

WILL: Don't know.

DAVID: You going to come back here again?

WILL: No way.

DAVID: Never?

WILL: Not for a long time anyway and then only once.

DAVID: You don't want to be here anyway. You've got your whole life in front of you. Haven't you? You should be out having a laugh, get yourself a girlfriend or something, not stuck up in here.

WILL: You're stuck in here.

DAVID: Yeh, but I go home at night. You don't. So have you thought about what you're going to do in the years to come?

WILL: Yes.

DAVID: Thought so. Copper?

WILL: No.

DAVID: Drug dealer?

WILL: No way.

DAVID: You going to be famous then?

WILL: Yeh.

DAVID: Write a movie or something?

WILL: That's right.

DAVID: Yeh good. That's it then. Get out of here! I never want to see you again unless it's when you're visiting. I'm on holiday as from tonight, you see.

Will gets up opens the door and hears David say his name and then say 'hardcore uproar' once more. Will smiles and carries on walking to see the girl of his dreams in the club of his dreams. Jacques Lacan could not make this scene anymore realistic. The MC is heard chanting "hardcore, you know the score". Will is now dressed up in his rave gear with cool shades on. He walks to where the girl is dancing. With his bare top half he walks next to her on the stage. He is just about to start dancing when she stops and gives him a massage. The melodic piano tune song of bye bye sugar pie is heard and Will is in ecstasy.

The room at the start of the film is shown again. Will is pouring two vodkas with black Russian. He gives one to his wife and says "alright Honey". It is the same girl that gave him the massage in the club.

CHAPTER 4

Madness in Greek Tragedy

I wanted to include the Dissertation I wrote at Manchester University whilst studying a BA (Hons) in Classical Studies (in 1998) in 'Curing Madness' to illustrate historical evidence that the madman has been alienated and suffered humiliation for thousands of years. In Ancient Greece to be mad was the ultimate punishment for hubris, even worse than death. This fact illustrates how the status quo has alienated mad people throughout history and seen them as evil. Recovery for the mentally ill is therefore made much more difficult because they see themselves as inferior as society gives them a raw deal. Unless you have been labelled with a psychiatric illness yourself or witnessed someone close to you who has it is very difficult to imagine the psychological damage this can have when someone attempts to rebuild their life after a breakdown.

"This dissertation is submitted in accordance with the regulations for the Part II examination in the Honours school of Classical Studies, University of Manchester".

1. INTRODUCTION

2. WHAT CONSTITUTES MADNESS IN GREEK TRAGEDY?

3. THE MADNESS OF ORESTES

4. THE MADNESS OF AJAX

5. THE MADNESS OF AGAVE

6. THE MADNESS OF HERAKLES

7. THE THEME OF MADNESS IN TRAGEDY

8. WHAT CONSTITUES MADNESS TODAY?

9. CONCLUSION

INTRODUCTION

Before focusing on madness in Greek Tragedy I shall discuss the phenomenon of the madman in general. If someone is driving down the road and a car pulls out in front of them that person might be inclined to refer to the other person as crazy, or a lunatic, or a madman. This is a matter-of-fact reference to madness. However, problems arise when people say things that they do not mean and when they judge something that they do not understand.

The driver that name calls is guilty of contributing to both of these problems. Firstly, he does not mean that the other driver is clinically insane although he literally says that he is. Secondly, and more importantly, who does he think he is in categorising somebody like that? Of course, he judges in a moment of anger but would not a real madman be upset in the way that he is viewed? Although he should he would probably not, for if he was mad at the time of hearing the remark he would view it differently than a sane man. Still the madman does not deserve derogatory remarks. For being mad is difficult enough as it is. The remark is not directed at the madman but it is an example of society's hostile view towards the insane.

Fortunately, seventeenth century France saw a revolution in society's treatment of the mad[6]. For the first time institutions were built exclusively for the mentally ill. The madman no longer always had to

---

[6] Michael Foucault discusses this in his study of "Madness and Civilisation" (1967).

share cells with criminals or suffer humiliation on the streets but joined others in safe houses for the mad.[7]

Psychiatry set about trying to find a cure for madness, for ancient Greek culture and modern societies generally accepted that there was something wrong with being mad. Madness is an undesirable state to be in, I have been there myself, and I know what it is like[8]. The madman is different from the sane man and whilst attitudes to madness are becoming less prejudiced, the mentally ill are still regarded as an enigma. The natural fear of being mad oneself is the reason for any hostile portrayal by a real person. In Tragedy any hostile portrayal is rectified as it induces pathos. Only in the last fifty years in Britain has attempted suicide not been a criminal offence. The only time mentally ill people seem to be discussed in the news is under extreme circumstances. They may have killed someone with a machete or have been brain damaged by taking the wrong kind of medication. Whilst the reports may point out that the patient was not looked after properly, the horrific events may be misinterpreted and force the viewer to misunderstand the madman. The Media give a chilling representation of the madman and so does Greek Tragedy. Of course, they do not aim to give a sympathetic account of the madman and there is no reason why they should except for a humanitarian one. Madness in the context of Greek Tragedy is fascinating and gives a revealing insight into the history of the insane.

---

[7] This interpretation in its generalisation leads Jacques Derrida to the conclusion that Foucault's attempt to identify the history of madness is an impossible task (Derrida and Deconstruction page 202).

[8] The author suffers from bipolar effective disorder, more commonly known as manic depression.

WHAT CONSTITUTES MADNESS IN GREEK TRAGEDY?

The thirty one Greek Tragedies that are extant from the thousand or so that were written are sufficient in quantity for a modern reader to be able to identify and define madness within the genre. Madness in Greek Tragedy is caused by an external force. Specifically a god brings about Madness in one of two ways. The god induces madness always as the punishment of an individual for their own hubris or the hubris of one of their relatives. Herakles is made mad by Hera, while Ajax is made mad by Athena. Once they are mad both victims lose the ability for rational thought. The madman is deluded and out of control, and does things that he would not normally do.

The madmen and women in Greek Tragedy are not aware of what they are doing but think that they are. When they recover from their frenzied state they regret what they have done. Terrible deeds are done by the madman, deeds that can only be those of someone that is out of their wits.

They cannot be forgiven and cannot forgive themselves for what they have done unwittingly. If they survive, then the experience will haunt them for the rest of their lives. If they do not, then the ordeal was simply too much.

Being mad itself is depicted as evil. Mad behaviour is led by demonic forces whether actions have justification or not. Orestes may kill his mother as a means of revenge. Different levels of madness are represented by playwrights. For example, Aeschylus makes the Furies only 'haunt' Orestes (Cite), whilst

Sophocles makes them drive Orestes mad (Cite). Whilst vengeance contributes to Orestes' state in Aeschylus and Ajax's state in the Ajax (Cite), Euripides goes further and makes madness entirely external. Agave has no reason to kill her son; she does so because she is possessed by some Bacchic frenzy.

The madman is perceived as having contracted some kind of terrible disease. This leads to ridicule and humiliation. Teucer and Ajax are characters who experience this. Still there is a positive aspect to the treatment of madness in Greek Tragedy. For example, the reference to the mad, being part of a divine language (Ajax L243f) as they are like a "frenzied god not a man" places the madman on a superhuman level. This simile refers to a state of existence that a normal human being cannot achieve. The presentation of the madman as something out of the ordinary and extraordinary is something which remains consistent throughout Tragedy.

The function of the madman in Tragedy in my view is to extend Aristotle's standard realms of catharsis. Madness is a very powerful concept and Aeschylus, Sophocles and Euripides all benefit from addressing the theme of madness. There is possibly nothing worse that man can experience and therefore madness is the perfect medium for tragedy. When Agave holds her son's head thinking it is the head of a lion the devastation that madness can bring makes the spectator's stomach crawl. She is completely oblivious to what she has done. Only a madman (or madwoman) can do such a thing, the most grotesque and shocking moments of Greek Tragedy take the form of the mad experience.

Despite a wonderment and awe that soon transforms itself into fear, hate and condemnation, there is an attempt to cure these mad folk. Cadmus manages to cure Agave from her madness and his actions are similar to those of modern psychiatric techniques.

Although there is pity for the characters it is often forgotten as the characters assume a different identity when they are mad. Their behaviour is unwitting and the state of frenzy takes away their humanity. An educated reader is able to distinguish between the representation of madness in a realistic and in a bad light. Tragedy consistently presents madness in a realistic light. It explores the vulnerability of those that are mad and those that are affected by it. It evokes the fundamental point that madness is an isolated as well as an altered state of mind. The coming in, and out of it, are separate from the moments of insanity.

There is frequently in Tragedy reference to characters before, during and after their madness. Madness is easier to identify if there is something to compare it to. The normally conscientious and heroic Herakles would of course not kill his children if he were sane. Mad behaviour in Greek Tragedy is so intense that it leaps out from the text. When Ajax mistakenly tortures sheep instead of men anyone in their right mind would realise that he is at that moment a madman.

There is no reason to focus on whether people in Tragedy are rightly or wrongly regarded and treated as mad. For constant moralising detracts from the facts. There is also no need always to try and determine what constitutes madness in Greek Tragedy for madness in a sense defines itself, and it is what it is as the gods demand or enforce it. A mortal cannot escape suffering and a madman is constantly regarded as being in an abominable state. The madman is physically repulsive[9]. He vomits black bile and has overbearing rage in his eyes.

Madness is the consequence of Hubris. This occurs when an individual or member of a character's family is punished by the gods for being too arrogant. Ajax rejects Athena's advice and is therefore made mad for being guilty of hubris. There is no arguing with this, it just happens. Madness is part of fate in Greek Tragedy. The madman has nowhere to run or hide. He cannot recall the frenzied state and when he escapes from it he will not consciously be able to get back to it[10]. Instead he has to cope with the trauma and the consequences of his actions. Some cope better than others. Depending on the situation some characters can recover from it, others are engulfed by it.

An analysis of four characters already mentioned Orestes, Ajax, Agave and Herakles will identify why each becomes mad, what they do exactly, and how they cope with being mad, as well as with what they have done.

---

[9] Ruth Padel in her book "In And Out Of Mind" is fascinated by the physical manifestations of the madman in Tragedy.

[10] The reference to a madman wishing to get back to the mad state is interesting for two reasons. Firstly a return to madness makes the madman forget the present. Secondly, in Tragedy madwomen are given godlike powers (Agave and the Maenads). Here lies the positive aspect to madness in Greek tragedy.

THE MADNESS OF ORESTES

Now follows the treatment of Orestes by Aeschylus and Euripides. Firstly, Aeschylus and the Libation Bearers: Electra claims that the recognition scene is madness as it causes so much pain (L211). Madness is always associated with some kind of pain. The traumatic state of Orestes is worsened by the Furies. As he kills his mother the Furies haunt the murderer. They are visible only to Orestes with their "eyes burning, grim brows working over you in the dark - the dark sword of the dead!" (L290). Although they avenge the death of Agamemnon, who is slain by Clytemnestra, their presentation is similar to that of Satan and his devil worshippers[11]. With such powerful enemies Orestes falls into the abyss. The theme of darkness which goes hand in hand with vengeance is part of what might constitute madness but not sufficient to make someone mad on his or her own. For example, the Orestes of Aeschylus is in a sense in the dark as he alone sees the Furies and enacts vengeance by killing Aegisthus but is able to maintain a sane mind.

Mad people are blind to what they do when they are mad. The leader tells Orestes that "The blood's still wet on your hands. It puts a kind of frenzy in you" (1055). Here is proof that the moment he kills his mother he is in a sense mad. This is not clear cut madness as Orestes does not lose consciousness of what he is doing. He does, however, hallucinate as the Furies are present in the text. So this shows that the character has one of the symptoms of madness. What

---

[11] Satan is a concept that is developed after the date of the text and is mentioned as an appropriate form of communication between ancient Greek Tragedy and the modern viewer.

else made him adhere to "this murderous hate, this Fury?" (1075). The house of Atreus is an infectious, disease ridden place. Orestes and his family are all victims of a curse put on them. This curse is contagious and Orestes catches its symptoms. For example, if his mother kills his father then vengeance demands Orestes to commit matricide.

In the Eumenides Orestes is cured. He is protected by Apollo who tells him to kill Clytemnestra (L200). Apollo drives back the Furies with his bow and arrows (175-8). Apollo says that the Furies' "manhunt of Orestes is unjust" (L219). Their pursuit of him multiplies their pains (L224).

It is the shrieking frenzy, the hymn of fury that causes pain to Orestes and the Furies themselves (L330 + L343). This hymn of fury as an external force is something that deities older than the gods cannot escape. Symptoms for the Furies are black froth erupting from their lungs (L180)[12]. There is no indication in Aeschylus where this suffering comes from except that it is fate punishing Orestes' grandfather Atreus (L1066LB). It is part of the curse on the house of Atreus. Still it is ultimately in the control of the new deities. The Gods rid Orestes of his torment as he has suffered enough. Orestes is the figure closest to being a madman that is explicitly treated and cured by the gods (L767Euminides). He is freed from guilt but is most definitely not mad in Aeschylus.

---

[12] Here Padel comments on the physical manifestations of the madman (throughout the text). Her categorising of all madmen having these physical attributes is misleading as Orestes in Aeschylus fits her definition of madness but is not actually mad. Her work exemplifies the danger of giving absolutes in critical theory.

The cure of Orestes lies in the need for the new judicial system to supplant that of the old. His recovery provides the mechanism to impose the Olympian gods ahead of the weary old deities, the furies, and with it come the law makers of torment. The law itself can be described as fate which supplies the origins of any manic or schizophrenic state for any character of Tragedy.

The Orestes of Euripides, however, is mad. He is punished with madness for slaying his mother (L37+400). Electra tells us this madness is "heaven-inflicted" (L844). He is pursued by the Furies, who are physically repulsive "gazing blood, horrid with snakes" (L256). Tyndarus points out that Orestes is "hated by the gods" for killing his mother (L531). He realises that it was "unholy" to slay his mother (L545). There are also suggestions that his madness is infectious when he speaks to Pylades, "take care how thou art partner of my madness" (L790).

The Orestes of Euripides is a character who is in need of more careful attention. His "grievous malady" (L36) causes him to lie at his sister's feet (L87). He is physically exhausted and weak (L228). He cannot control his madness that comes in fits (L227). He was deluded by the gods when slaying Helen (L1589). His eyes roll when he raves with madness (L839). This Orestes is madder than in Aeschylus. His madness is infectious and incurable. He kills Clytemnestra and Helen and is only just prevented from killing Hermione. Apollo's forcing of Orestes to marry Hermione does not cure him from madness for he still suffers (L1681). The god enacts destiny

(L1654), and although Orestes has a future there is no indication that he is relieved from his madness.

The chorus want the madness to stop (L332-3) as they want the suffering to stop in the Libation Bearers (1067f). They are unable to do anything about it. Insanity corrupts men as does war and comes from within. Only the gods can enforce it. This makes the suffering of the madman and those observing him more tragic as they are helpless to prevent what is inevitable.

Orestes borders on madness as he is always haunted by the Furies. Their sick and frenzied hounding is sufficient to make any mortal question his or her sanity. Orestes is never in control of his actions. He may have a justified reason for killing his mother but he is ultimately an unwitting contributor to fate. His appearance borders on the schizophrenic[13], with delusions and the witnessing of horrible evil creatures suffocating his existence. In Aeschylus and Euripides his relation to other people in the text is symptomatic of a schizophrenic as only he has delusions.

As Cassandra is the misunderstood prophet, Orestes alone suffers from the wrath of the Furies. He has nowhere to run or hide. Within the conventions of Greek Tragedy his character's suffering produces catharsis and adds to plot detail. In Euripides he can be said to have had a horrific mental breakdown caused by external circumstance. For other characters within the play cannot see the Furies and do not understand what Orestes is going through. His ability

---

[13] Medical conditions were not recognised in the same way in ancient Greek culture as they are by some today, but the work of Euripides inevitably evokes comparisons with modern illnesses.

to maintain consciousness despite the persistent harping of the Furies reveals him to be a character that is mentally strong and resilient.

However, the damage is already done. Vengeance forces him to kill his mother and he will never recover from this terrible crime. Like Oedipus he commits matricide which is one of the worst crimes imaginable (L886LibationBearers). Apollo possesses him in order to carry out the matricide as he could not do it with a sane mind. His family is not exempt from hubris, however. The House of Atreus is damned by the gods when Thyestes eats his children. They carry out the fate of Orestes.

He is motivated by the external force that he can never control. He discovers that Apollo made him kill his mother only after he has done it. Still, if he had known at the time of the event what he was doing resistance to the will of Apollo would have been equally futile. Of course he has a certain justification for committing matricide so may not have wished to refrain if he had been sane. This identifies a problem with discussing insanity which is that it drives one into moral speculation as it is such a powerful subject.

All mortals in Greek Tragedy have to bow to the superior gods. The problem for the Orestes of Euripides is that his submission to the external force allows madness to come to the fore. He is released from his madness. Orestes could have been permanently insane or killed himself. The conventions of Greek Tragedy, uses madness for its own means. It explores the consequences, causes, nature and modes of madness as it sees fit. As regards to the madness of Euripides' Orestes, he withstands it, is given it, is not responsible for it and experiences different types of it. He is a victim of demonic forces that are part of an unjust world. His response to it is a brave one and to be admired.

Euripides continued the treatment of Orestes where Aeschylus left off. Euripides made his Orestes mad and by doing so induced more suffering and pathos in his treatment.

THE MADNESS OF AJAX

The Ajax of Sophocles describes a madman who cannot cope with the consequences of his madness. Ajax is so disturbed at having been mad that he stabs himself to death (L866). He leaves his family and friends behind (L855). Humiliation is the reason for his suicide. He says "look at my shame" (L366) and "I am their laughing stock" (L455). Ajax feels that all of Greece will laugh at him for killing sheep when he meant to kill Agamemnon and his company. This would qualify him as a paranoid schizophrenic today. He suffers from hallucinations and fears the worst possible scenario which is suicide.

In course of the play Ajax loses his heroic code of honour. The tragic hero must "bring back honour for my father". His failure to win Achilles' belt and act of hubris make suicide his only way to "die with honour" (L478). His suicide will show his bravery and restore him to the heroic hall of fame.
Unlike Orestes, Ajax is guilty of hubris. He tells Athena:

I'll do anything you ask - except change my plans for Odysseus.

Athena appears to accept what Ajax says but we already know that she has "warped his sight". She hates him as he "thought himself an equal of the Gods" (L777). As the paranoid schizophrenic when depressed would feel that he is an embarrassment to society because he has manic thoughts and delusions,[14] Ajax must be made to feel the same way for his inflated

---

[14] The author comes to this conclusion based on patients that he has met in various mental institutions.

opinion of himself[15]. He is not a god, only a mortal that is too arrogant for his own good. He has offended those that are superior to him so must be punished in a fitting manner. He is made an example of. "Athena's broken toy" (401) makes a slaughter house full of sheep instead of men (L55). To effect his humiliation Athena turns his brain with wild thoughts of revenge (L51).

As with Agave, Tecmessa gives a fascinating insight on madness. She says of Ajax that he was happier when he was mad (L270). The trauma of coping with the actions of his madness is too much to bear. The moments of madness themselves are enjoyable although they are disfunctional. Ajax is happy as long as he maintains madness. As soon as he comes out of it he is forced to face the real world and deal with the terrible events of his madness. Ajax is not given the opportunity to deal only with returning to reality. With madness regarded as a terrible affliction he will always blame his madness for the predicament that he is in (which is of course true). However, he does not deny it but faces up to it immediately, for Ajax is no coward but is a man of bravery. His tragedy is that through being mad he has lost his honour.

Only madness could have driven him to do such things (L181). Madness even induces fear in one of the most intelligent and caring characters in the whole of Greek Tragedy. Odysseus tells Athena that he will not face the madman (L82).

---

[15] Simon Bennett "Mind and Madness in Ancient Greece" (p93) refers to divine agencies driving the protagonist mad. This provides the most humane treatment of Madness (of all the texts that I have read on madness in Greek Tragedy)

Poor Ajax is left in limbo. What can he do? He feels that society is against him. He feels that the gods are against him. People do not understand what he has been through. Once one of the noblest of the Greeks, he loses so much dignity that he chooses to end his life. His suicide is presented as brave and tragic. There are no gods on his side. He leaves his wife, son and comrades, whom he loves very much. He refuses to ask for any sympathy. Instead he goes quietly and takes his own life. Brave in life and brave in death (L1337). The one flaw of hubris is sufficient to destroy him and devastate those that are close to him.

The Herakles in Euripides' Herakles manages to live on after realising that he has killed his children. He has divine help, unlike Ajax. The suggestion that there is honour in suicide is extraordinarily advanced in my view[16]: As recently as in the early twentieth century suicide was a criminal offence and frequently viewed as the 'easy way out'. People are as scared of suicide and madness today as they were in Greek tragedy. This is why they condemn it. In Ajax suicide is his decision and is part of his destiny.

Madness instigates his suicide. The madness is external, although he unwittingly contributes to it. His ordeal demonstrates man's powerlessness against fate. This is also true in Oedipus Tyrannus, where patricide and marrying one's mother is inevitable. Ajax's pride makes him succumb to the wrath of Athena. His choice of suicide is a way of the tragedian

---

[16] Large sections of modern culture view suicide as a cowardly act. See the final act of the play Hedda Gabler by Henrik Ibsen. Throughout the play the motives for and reaction to suicide are the underlying themes. Hedda shoots herself in the final act like Ajax because she feels trapped. She chooses suicide as her escape.

characterising Ajax as somebody who cannot cope with madness. As victim of overbearing external forces and traumatic circumstances his suicide is realistic.

Others suffer from Ajax's madness. Teucer is ridiculed, spat at, harrassed and threatened for being the "brother of a madman and a traitor" (L720f). The chorus of the followers of Ajax when discovering his death are so upset that they might as well be dead (L900). As Ajax is no longer there to protect them Tecmessa worries that she and her son will be slaves to Agamemnon (L944).

The situation when Ajax has recovered from his madness is significant as it shows the damage which mad behaviour can cause. It suggests two paradoxes, either that the madman is not alone but feels he is, or that he is alone and does not feel like he is. For example, Ajax kills himself since he feels he is alone, but in fact his family and friends are in a sense with him. They are on his side. If his family is not with him he imagines people to be ridiculing him.

Sophocles has presented madness and its consequences in a realistic manner which is similar to modern psychiatric thought. Ajax unfortunately refuses to treat himself so that he can recover. Odysseus gives back Ajax some dignity by saving his burial rights. Having a proper burial is an essential part of showing respect to those who have died in ancient Greek culture.

Tecmessa's references to Ajax being possessed (L218) and acting like a "frenzied god" are reminiscent of the constant hounding that Orestes had to endure. The chorus do not know whether Ajax is mad again or whether he is horrified at what his madness has done to him (L337). They soon discover it is the latter. The madness of Ajax is more damaging than that of Euripides' Orestes as it leads ultimately to death. Orestes' madness comes in fits and is equally as traumatic, but it is managed. With the actions of madness that Ajax has done his loyalty to the heroic code makes him kill himself. Society would say his fate is tragic. Existentialists could argue that Ajax is lucky to escape a finite existence and obtain the inevitability of death[17].

Whatever interpretation is held regarding the fate of Ajax, he is a tragic hero whose pride is his weakness. This weakness is the reason for his suffering in the play. His madness is the consequence of his act of hubris. Odysseus finds a way to save his reputation but Ajax still remains notoriously mad. Pride is a fault of all men though, and Athena's victim is merely privy to fate which determines the action of the goddess. As if it were a disease, madness engulfs him and he is unable to prevent it from ruining him.

The character of Ajax presents a realistic response to madness. It is so powerful that nobody is able to cope with what it does. There is no necessity to speculate what kind of madness Ajax suffers from as these diagnoses are neither part of Greek Tragedy nor ancient Greek culture. However, he can be described as being on a high one minute and then on a low the next. This pattern of behaviour is similar to that of the manic depressive. Many kinds of mental illness can induce this kind of dysfunctional behaviour. As soon as

---

[17] Jean Paul Sartre is, as far as I know, the pioneer of thought expressed in this manner. This view derives from the reading of Speech and Language in Psychoanalysis by Jacques Lacan.

Ajax is out of his mind he is recognisably mad and when he is in his mind he is sane.[18] Therefore Ajax fails to manage the illness that inflicts him.

Sophocles demonstrates the worst possible scenario that madness causes. Madness is so overpowering that it can lead a hero to commit suicide. This is where Sophocles' treatment of madness is unique.

All other madmen in Greek Tragedy survive to mourn the consequences of their mad actions. Bearing this in mind, it becomes frustrating that hundreds of Greek Tragedies are missing. With the plays that have been restored Sophocles and not Euripides deals with the suicide of a madman. The reputation of Euripides as a radical Tragedian therefore is not merely because he chooses the most disastrous consequences of madness.

Sophocles also chooses not to describe Ajax coming out of his madness. This is a significant difference from Euripides, who analyses the recovery of Herakles and Agave very closely.

---

[18] Here the title of Ruth Padel's book "In and Out of Mind" is the most appropriate language for losing and recovering one's sanity.

THE MADNESS OF AGAVE

There is no doubt that the visual images of the madman (madwoman in this case) in the Bacchae of Euripides are the most disturbing in the whole of Greek tragedy[19]. How is a mother to react when she realises that she has hunted her son and holds his head and not that of a lion? If she loves her son as Agave clearly does she will be devastated (L1279-1288). Killing one's child is at the very least equally disturbing for Agave as the matricide of Orestes. It is possibly more disturbing for Agave as she has no motive for killing her son unlike the vengeful Orestes. The viewer is voyeur of much more graphic detail than the murder itself (in the Bacchae). This naturally adds to the visual effect in the play and induces more pathos.

She cannot remember her actions during the Bacchic frenzy (L1294-5). Madness is a punishment for slandering and ultimately causing the death of Semele, the mother of Dionysus (L1297). Agave and her sisters are made mad as a means of revenge for Dionysus (L26).

Ajax's acceptance of Athena as a deity shows that Sophocles does not go as far as Euripides. Regarding the treatment of madness, Euripides makes the denial of Dionysus the act of hubris. Pentheus had no idea that Dionysus was a god. The fate of Pentheus is grim because he refuses to worship Dionysus (L44). The play shows the prevailing theme that humans are

---

[19] I disagree with Bennett (M&Mp124f), who believes that *Ajax* is the most visual treatment of madness. Ajax is unique in that he kills himself, but there is no imagery as powerful as Agave holding aloft the head of her son or ripping his body apart in the *Ajax*.

powerless to prevent the punishment that a god enacts.

The consequences of Agave's madness are that she will be parted from her father (L1363) and forced into exile (1368). So madness is once again responsible for isolating individuals and is portrayed as a contagious disease that nobody in their right mind wants to catch. Pentheus catches the disease and can only then die from it. Agave's response to having killed Pentheus is in my view rather abrupt[20]. The lines after her realisation are sadly missing (L1301f). Still she is clearly in untold grief, mourning, disbelief and horror at what she has done (L1279-88).

Agave is not to blame for her mad actions as she did them unwittingly. She is responsible for offending Dionysus but is human and therefore prone to make mistakes. The mad episode has totally ruined her life. She must seek another identity elsewhere for her act of hubris. Her punishment is too severe as Dionysus agrees (L1347).

However, Zeus is described as ordaining that offending the gods makes the punishment suitable if not desirable (L1348).

As a result of her madness Cadmus and her sisters must be exiled (L1352). Pentheus cannot be given a respectable funeral. Although there is a lacuna after lines 1300, the previous line describes Agave asking whether the body is torn limb from limb or not? The answer is most definitely yes. There is a detailed scene earlier that shows how the body of Pentheus is ripped

---

[20] What she does to Pentheus is so tragic that the subject could cover an entire play.

to pieces. She grabs his left arm, places her foot against his ribs and tears his shoulder out of its socket (1127).

Agave has graver consequences to deal with than the quick stabbing of Orestes or the torturing of sheep of Ajax. She has to deal with the fact that she kills her son, tortures him, holds his head apart from its body and rips his whole body to shreds. This is a disgusting thought, nauseous to anyone in their right mind, and can only be performed by someone who is out of their mind. However, each madman has their own problems to face; Orestes has the Furies haunting him, whilst Ajax has his heroic honour amongst other things to consider.

All Agave's suffering derives from offending Dionysus and the gods. For denying that Dionysus is a god (L45) he makes the women involved mad by joining in Bacchanal worship (L32). This frenzy singles out Agave amongst the women who refuse to worship and pour libations to the god. When Dionysus says that he will reveal himself as a god (L47) this is an indication that hell will break loose.

The prologue makes it quite clear that Dionysus' principal victim is Pentheus (L47). Throughout the text there are warnings that you must "honour the gods" (L1010) otherwise you will be "stung by madness by Dionysus" (L118). The play explores Pentheus changing from a sane character to a character who is mad. Dionysus invades his personality making him see the god turn into a bull as he tries to lock him up. The Bacchae is unique in tragedy as the treatment of Pentheus and Dionysus provides the only extensive interaction between the agency and the victim of madness[21]. This interaction shows that Dionysus is an embodiment of the unconscious impulses and fears of Pentheus[22]. For example, the dress making scene describes the god encouraging the manly Pentheus to dress up as a woman so that he can view the worship of the Maenads (L810f). The man who could not put on female garb (L836) has his mind altered by the god and becomes fascinated by how he looks when he is dressed as a woman. He wonders whether he looks like his mother (L924) and notices if a curl is out of place (L930). Pentheus is clearly mad at this point as he sees "two suns and a double Thebes" (L918) and Dionysus as a bull (L920). The presentation of Pentheus emphasizes that in madness delusion is accompanied by a blurring of the self and the other, a confusion of personal identity.

Teiresias says that a man is a bad citizen if he lacks sanity (L271). This comment suggests that madness is an undesirable state abhorred by those in their right mind. The mad Bacchanals are a terrifying bunch with their cries of ecstasy (L149 + L156). Pentheus is terrified at the thought of being caught by them. However, more significantly, Teiresias notices that "that which is manic possesses great mantic powers". This introduces a positive element of madness within the play. The messenger's speech describes the quiet of the Bacchic women and their peaceful occupations (L677-774). The madness of Agave is consistent in the psychological order in which the madness of Pentheus is described and has a different emphasis. She too is driven mad by Dionysus but by absorption into the Maenads as opposed to personal interaction with the god. The Maenads are

---

[21] See Simon Bennett, Mind & Madness, pages 115-116.
[22] See Simon Bennett, Mind & Madness, pages 113-122.

able to express their femininity by worshipping Dionysus when they nurse young animals. They are more powerful than armed men with their thyrsoi but as the thiasos revolves around a male leader they lack penis power and the prerogatives of men[23]. Pentheus breaks down because he is unable to accept a feminine side of himself that lacks power (L310); the women are dependant upon a male no matter how effeminate he may be. Therefore group ecstasy becomes madness because the Bacchic ecstasy does not resolve underlying conflict. The theme of group madness is exclusive to the Bacchae.

The Maenads are presented as perfectly peaceful and in harmony with nature until they are interfered with. Dionysus gives the Bacchanals great strength. How else can they pull a huge tree out of the ground? (L1110). These women drink honey and milk, wear fawnskins, hissing snakes and hold clubs. They attack everything they see when they are in a state of frenzy. Their behaviour is due to their denial of Dionysus and therefore because of their hubris. They are the tools of his vengeance.

The good sense of Teiresias is shown when he refuses the demands of Pentheus and the chorus to go against the god:

For you are most grievously mad - beyond the cure of drugs, and yet your sickness must be due to them (L326-7)

Teiresias knows that you should not "raise arms against a god" (L789). He realises that the gods are better than mortals and he will never be guilty of

---

[23] See Simon Bennett, Mind & Madness page 119.

hubris. His behaviour demonstrates that madness is a grim state that nobody wishes to experience. He would be of the opinion that once Pentheus is mad he is doomed (L44). Dionysus is the instigator (L305) and is directly responsible for the suffering of the mad Pentheus and Agave. Dionysus claims that he follows the law of his father Zeus who has to carry out fate as it is set out before him (L1348). This shows Dionysus on the defensive as he shifts responsibility onto Zeus in order to rid himself of guilt. This behaviour exemplifies the presentation of Dionysus as an imperfect god in the play. It also reveals that Euripides is more critical of the gods in their enforcement of madness than Sophocles.

Agave suffers from various types of madness, although Greek Tragedy does not distinguish between them. Her mood is high when she joins in the festivities of the Bacchanals only for her mood to be lowered when she comes out of the manic state[24]. The events of the Bacchae show that tragic events are problems that mortals have to deal with. The play criticises the god's handling of madness as a punishment implying that it is too severe. It incorporates positive and negative aspects of madness in a realistic manner.

---

[24] The use of modern terminology of high and low mood is expanded here from the earlier discussion on Ajax.

THE MADNESS OF HERAKLES

There is no explicit reference that madness will invade Herakles until Iris speaks (L823). Herakles is not mad until the second half of the play. Madness is so powerful that time is of little significance in inducing pathos upon the plight of a madman. Sophocles makes Ajax dead half way through the play whilst Euripides makes Agave mad throughout the Bacchae. Each play has its own style in presenting madness. However, the mad appearance of Herakles is the central theme of the play.

No other mad tragic figure except Herakles kills his wife and offspring. Is there anything more precious to a man than the well being of his wife and children? Will his removal of them all show his world falling apart? Will he end up like Ajax? Yes, yes and no respectively. He suffers great torment for what he has done but lives to tell the tale.

Facing up to the murder of his wife and three children are the immediate consequences of the madness of Herakles. These catastrophes are presented in a way worse than that which Orestes and Ajax have to endure, and are on a par with the devastated Agave, for Herakles kills more than one person that he loves. He feels responsible for murdering four of the closest people to him. Before the murders sympathy is increased for Herakles when he mentions that everyone adores children (L638). The misery that his madness induces also satisfies the wrath of Hera (L830) and resolves her vengeance.

The main problem for Herakles is trying to cope with what he has done. His father has to point out the terrible deeds, as the murderer has no idea what he has done when he first comes out of the frenzied state. The response of Herakles is one of total anguish (L1132). He asks whether he was possessed or if it was his own doing (L1142). Either way his first thought when he realises the effect of what he has done, is to kill himself (L1147). Like Ajax he contemplates suicide and hides himself in shame at the terrible atrocities that his madness has done (L1159). It is mostly the remarkable loyalty of Theseus but also that of his father which makes Herakles choose to live (L1219 + 1399). Ajax has the support of the chorus and his family but is unable to step out from his responsibilities under the heroic code.

Thanks to the loyalty of his friend, Herakles is able to stand although his limbs have seized up (L1396). This pathetic moment reveals a realistic cure to someone who is mad. In effect, good friends can help you conquer the terrible affliction. This emphasis is specifically Euripidean. Amphtryion helps Herakles as Cadmus helps Agave come to terms with the consequences of her madness. Sophocles does not attempt to bring Ajax out of madness directly but instead makes Tecmessa describe his recovery (L306f). Euripides' treatment of Herakles choosing to live on avoiding suicide is a fundamental concept of psychotherapy[25]. However, in Greek Tragedy madness has already left Herakles enabling him to recover.

---

[25] Shirley Barlow presents this phenomenon in her introduction on Herakles 1996. Its relevance here is not to challenge that the madness of Herakles is enacted as is always the case in tragedy by *hubris* but to make the modern psychiatric point that chemical conditions and psychological states are both equally significant causes of mental illness.

Herakles is not responsible for the murders as they stem from the madness that is inflicted upon him (L1187). He knows himself that he is hated by Hera (L1264). His denial of what Zeus is, is the reason for carrying out labours and rebuttal of him as his father shows that the man whom Amphitryon hails as being as capable of saving his family as his godly father is guilty of hubris.

He has the curse of the Furies (L1077) like Orestes. He celebrates his madness in a similar way to Agave in the Bacchae. He rejoices in Bacchic ritual dancing to the mad frenzy of the pipe (L878). The Bacchic madness is so strong (L898) that he is only freed from it by being physically knocked out by Athena (L1005). The chorus tell us that the madness is fated (L1024) and Iris reveals that Hera is responsible. The law of gods makes certain that Hera's anger will be felt by Herakles. Only by this treatment can gods show that they are superior to mortals (L840). Fate comes before Hera's decision for vengeance. Nobody is responsible. The spectator knows that madness occurs from within Tragedy.

Fate dominates the cause and nature of madness. Madness is a form of punishment. Madmen have no control whether they are mad or not. Herakles is punished but his character is strong enough to survive it. He passes the test that a god lays out in front of him where Ajax fails. The first episode of Herakles coincides with the murders whilst his emphatic recovery is the end of his madness.

His mad episode is an unwitting one. Lyssa points out that he will not realise that he has killed his children until her madness leaves him (L863). The nature of his madness is so upsetting that she remarks how she is against it (L858). This sympathy from a god is exclusive to the Herakles. Apollo in the Orestes shows a little sympathy for mankind in preventing Orestes from committing another murder but this is ultimately so he can be worshipped. Herakles is privy to the actions of Lyssa, she must follow the law set by Hera who enacts fate for Zeus. Herakles suffers in similar ways to Orestes, Ajax and Agave. His eyes are poisoned (L866) and froth falls out of his mouth (L934). He hallucinates believing that his children are those of Eurystheus (L969).

He is not in his right mind. He has had a history of mental anguish, for he has not only had to endure the ten labours which would drive any sane man wild but also when he was only a baby Hera sent frightening serpents to kill him (L1266). His madness is so intense that on his return from it he is not sure who is his father nor is he familiar with anything at all (L1106). It pollutes him and those around him (L1398). The fact that madness can make a man who has been to Hades and killed the dreaded Cerberus (L609) wish to turn himself into stone (L1395) shows how vulnerable mortals are.

The essence of Tragedy makes it inevitable that it is a nightmarish event which constitutes his madness. Herakles becomes deranged as soon as the gods enforce it. He has no awareness or control over what his madness does. He shows every aspect of the deranged mental asylum archetype. He is off his head, loony and a nutter. He enjoys the experience giving a maniacal laugh (L935). This shows a solitary positive aspect to his madness. His state of delusion at this moment in the text is enjoyable; however, it does not compensate for the ensuing horrific consequences of the experience. He wrestles with people that are not there (L959). His madness is so intense that it takes a violent strike by Athena with a stone to rid him of it.

His return from madness guides him through what has happened to him and makes him face up to it. It is realistic and is a pioneer for modern Clinical Psychology. The questions Herakles raises about what constitutes his madness are answered and put into context by Amphitryion. In this way he is guided back into accepting what he has done to his family. All the madmen and women in Tragedy are released from madness once their punishment is complete. The characters of Euripides cope with the aftermath of madness better than the characters of anyone else. It is not my prerogative to discuss whether the characters of Euripides reach higher levels of madness or are the most resourceful in tragedy but Agave and Herakles are certainly thicker skinned than Ajax.

THE THEME OF MADNESS IN TRAGEDY

Always as a form of punishment madness is immediately recognised as something that is bad for you. It is therefore an undesirable state. Just as a Christian fears Hell the characters of Tragedy are terrified of what madness induces individuals to do (L261Ajax). Madmen are not blamed for what they have done. For example the chorus in Ajax mourn the suicide of Ajax and claim that they might as well die with him (L900). Also in the Bacchae, Agave tears Pentheus to pieces but she is not blamed by her father for killing his grandson. Cadmus feels deep grief for his daughter (L1217) and assists her to come out of her madness (L1277). Madness is such a powerful medium in Tragedy that it tears people apart and brings people together in mourning.

The Tragedians utilise madness as a powerful theme to induce empathy for their characters and the society that they write about as a whole. Characters are sometimes more tragic if they appear to be mad. Therefore Tragedy is frequently more powerful if it explores madness. What can be more tragic for the spectator than seeing the actor's world destroyed by the actor? The answer is nothing as the involvement of the spectator does not go any further than empathy for the actor. The question also elucidates the all - important Aristotelian distinction between the spectator and actor - we see someone else seeing himself destroying his own world. The actor is not in control of his actions and neither is the character especially when he is mad.

The madman feels guilt as he feels responsible for his actions. However his mad actions stem from hubris which is part of fate. The gods punish the relations of an individual if they do not wish merely to condemn the guilty party. For example Herakles is wounded by the gods as a child and he is not made mad because of hubris. The vengeance of Hera is the reason for his psychotic frenzy which is part of his destiny. Even the goddess herself serves Zeus. Zeus may have ordained that mortals are to be punished if they have unsettled the gods but he can only postpone fate not change it.

Characters that commit acts such as hubris do so because they make mistakes. As they are mortal they will keep on making mistakes. The characters' behaviour, identity, beliefs and actions are only consistent in their inconsistency. The only thing consistent about the madman in Tragedy is that he suffers tremendous pain. The inevitability of grief and death in Tragedy evokes what is an almost existentialist ideology. As the Greeks did not believe in the after-life in the fifth century BC this is a remarkably advanced perception within Tragedy. The existentialist comparison is more suitable to Tragedy than elsewhere in Greek literature. There is no time for the hero dying the heroic death as Hector does in the Iliad and for him to perform heroic tasks within Tragedy as it explores the characters' identities and sufferings in such a profound manner. The serious nature of Tragedy urges the spectator to think and reflect on telling circumstances.

What better way is there to show characters suffering than through madness? There is no better way as madness is unique in presenting characters that suffer. It makes them do things that the sane person would not even dream of doing and also makes them deal with the consequences of their actions.

Modern metaphors of madness such as Hell and the abyss add to the curiosity of what it is like to be mad. An analysis of the happy delusions of Ajax torturing Agamemnon's men and Agave's celebrations at slaughtering Pentheus show that the moments of madness themselves are not undesirable. When a character returns from the abyss they can not believe what they have done and have no way of changing it. By causing such regret in the character the author is able to manipulate the emotions of the spectator.

There are notable distinctions between Greek Tragedians. Sophocles omits Ajax coming out of madness and makes Athena describe it instead (L306). This shows the horror that madness can cause both the character and the spectator. Euripides deals with it directly in detail slowly bringing Herakles back into the real world via dialogue (L1106f) and Agave likewise (L1277). Sophocles' treatment lacks the psychological advances of the later fifth century BC. Although it was produced earlier than Aeschylus' Oresteia (458BC) the Ajax (mid440sBC) comes before the teaching of rhetoric of Gorgias (427BC). As one of the pioneers of Sophistry Gorgias sought expediency of action and denied the absolute moral actions of the earlier part of the fifth century[26]. Euripides benefits from the likes of Gorgias as Herakles (430-420BC) and the Bacchae (406BC) were produced during the first generations of Sophistic thought. As the seminal figure of epistemology Gorgias' thoughts are evoked in Euripides' text. How do Agave and Herakles know that they are mad? They have to be told in stages by

---

[26] See Greece and Rome *The Birth of Western Civilization* page 83.

Cadmus and Amphitryion. The moment when they realise that they are or have been mad they recover from their madness. For this reason Euripides' treatment of madness is the most sophisticated of the Greek Tragedians.

There are parameters to madness in Greek Tragedy. Fate carries out what happens and madness fits within this context. The madness of characters in Tragedy is presented with empathy and pathos and each individual is cured. Herakles avoids permanently remaining mad which is a bloody pollution (L1398) and when cured goes into exile. This evokes the humiliating fate for distinguished people in Ancient Greece as does the exile of Agave. For characters of such noble background as Agave and Herakles exile is a tragic outcome.

Only several of the thirty-one remaining plays use the theme of madness in depth. There are other plays that come close to inducing madness on their characters. The experiences of Deianera in Sophocles' Women of Trachis and Electra in Electra are both so distressing that they border on madness but they do not fit the criteria for madness as they are not guilty of hubris which means that they are not made mad as a punishment by a god. Their characters therefore lack the intensity which madness gives to a character such as Agave.

Madness is always presented as a form of divine influence that creates violence. As violence is a fundamental part of madness and its effects the tragedian is able to use it to impose a greater dramatic effect on the spectator.

Madmen are cured and helped when they return from their madness throughout Greek Tragedy. Orestes is pardoned (In Aeschylus) and has Menelaus for company (Euripides). Agave can go into exile with her sisters. Herakles is looked after by Theseus. Even Ajax comes out of his madness and is helped by Tecmessa and the chorus. Although he dies he receives a proper burial which salvages his reputation within the context of an ancient Greek culture. The brain of the mad character is permanently altered but this is what constitutes the best Tragedy.

Madness is presented as part of fate for individuals who have gone against the rites of a god. The behaviour of the mad character is inevitable and it is unfitting to draw their actions into moral speculation. For the mad character does things as he does them not because he should do them. It is also inevitable that the madman cannot be presented and received in a completely objective fashion. This draws critics into speculation, such as whether it is right that Orestes should be deprived of his humanity in Euripides' play. [27]

All the characters of Tragedy carry some of the same symptoms. Delusions, manic states, racy thoughts, depression, violent outbursts and paranoia. [28] They all contemplate suicide although Ajax is the only one that goes ahead with it. He suffers in a specific

---

[27] This is an assertion openly made by T.A. Buckley in his introduction to the translation of Euripides in 1887 and exemplifies the arid moral speculation of critics prior to modern deconstructive theory.

[28] These symptoms are identical to those experienced by sufferers of bipolar effective disorder today emphasizing that the presentation of madness in Tragedy is realistic.

way as does each character of the same attire. Madness occurs due to reasons outside of the individual's control. Only in the aftermath does the actor deal with it as the spectator tries to digest the text.

WHAT CONSTITUES MADNESS TODAY?

As the presentation of madness in Greek Tragedy is realistic what constitutes madness today is essentially the same as what it constitutes in Greek Tragedy. The difference lies in that madness in Greek Tragedy is governed by a law. In tragedy madness has a starting point and finishing point that is determined by a god. Madness today is identified as deriving from a combination of a chemical or psychological origin and we can only speculate on the nature of madness. For example bipolar effective disorder is believed to occur due to a lack of salt in the blood. When Lithium is taken as requested to counter-act the salt deficiency the individual concerned may still suffer from manic episodes. Therefore Psychotherapy searches for any destructive part of the individual's past that might be deemed as a contributor to their madness so that they can change the behaviour of the individual in a positive manner in order to remain sane.

Madness today is also categorised into different types of madness. There is no schizophrenic, manic depressive or psychotic in tragedy. Psychological advances in the last two and a half thousand years provide new interpretations on the texts (Herakles and the Bacchae) where Herakles and Agave are talked out of their madness by Amphitryion and Cadmus. Although there are different presentations of madness in Tragedy the dramatists do not distinguish between different types.[29] Herakles is recognisably mad as a

---

[29] There is no attempt to assimilate modern types of madness to characters in Greek Tragedy here as it is not entirely appropriate modern types of madness are not within the text.

character whether one describes him as a madman or a particular kind of madman. For madness, is as easily identified today, as it is in Tragedy.

The madman is defined by stereotypes. When Jack Nicholson walks into the dormitory near the end of "One Flew Over the Cuckoos Nest" having been lobotomised with his mouth wide open, eyes contorted, arms aloft and shaking his head from side to side, he has the same symptoms as a madman in Tragedy. Today, as it is in Tragedy, anything that is undesirable and not the doing of a sane man is the action of a madman.

The madman today may become the chronic patient of a mental asylum. There is no such safe house for the madman of Tragedy and no such place in Ancient Greek culture.[30] There is therefore a greater recognition today that the madman needs help. However, characters like Cadmus and Amphitryion in Tragedy are clearly sympathetic and assist those who are mad.

As the madman's mind leaves him he is excluded from the society which he is part of. Throughout history the madman has been abandoned. Ships from England would take mad people in boats to Australia in exile of them. The criminal was abandoned and left on his own for months as a punishment to see if solitude would drive him mad. The madman's identity remains a taboo

---

[30] If any critical text would mention the existence of mental asylums in ancient Greece it would be The Greeks and the Irrational and it does not. This book is the main influence on modern discussions of madness in Greek Tragedy. In my view its style lacks the critical accuracy of modern literary thought.

subject, or cause for ridicule. This kind of hostility towards the madman stems from the fear of being mad oneself.

A madman stands out from the convention of society whilst he is mad as this is the very essence of madness. He is out of his wits and unable to communicate with others in a world of his own. Tragedy explores madness in the same way and also identifies the parameters in which the madman will behave. It explains that madness is the dark side of man's mortality and the role of madness has not changed today.

CONCLUSION

It is a basic premise of Tragedy and ancient Greek culture in general that no-one can handle the experience of madness. It is also a prime function of Tragedy to enable at least an approximation to emotive identification with people of different experience. This function as regards to the experience of madness is best carried out by Euripides. Aeschylus does not actually misunderstand[31] and Sophocles understands exactly what madness makes a character do but neither can provide an effective positive aspect to it. It is only Herakles and Agave that are nurtured out of their madness. These pathetic moments represent the basis of modern treatments of Psychotherapy and confirm Euripides as the superior poet on the theme of madness in Greek Tragedy.

Those who are mad in Tragedy are possessed by an undesirable state. Characters kill themselves, their wives, mothers and children because of madness. The presentation of such terrible events invites the spectator to interpret that the madman needs to be sympathised with if not cared for. Their physical disabilities of sight, foaming at the mouth and seizures present accurately the horrors of being mad. However, the most painful part of the mad experience is coming out of it. This is precisely what is demonstrated in the Bacchae when Agave is holding the head of her son. The fact that Sophocles does not describe Ajax coming out of madness directly is the most striking difference between him and Euripides.[32]

---

[31] This judgement of Aeschylus is because, as stated earlier, none of his character's not even Orestes are mad.

All three dramatists are capable of powerful visualisation in their plays. Ajax butchers sheep and falls on his own sword alone on the sea shore. This is a visual play but lacks the same intensity as Agave and her colleagues tearing her son to pieces then celebrating waving her son's head around bereft of its body.

There are moments of great physical strength during mad episodes. The Maenads ripping a huge tree from out of the ground show godlike strength (L1109). Although this is used in a violent way it represents a positive aspect of madness. Madness allows a character to have the power of a god for a short time. It provides a temporary escape from mortality before the damage it causes is realised by the instigator. The reactions of Cadmus and Amphitryion are remarkable. They show no bitterness towards the murderers as they are loyal and realise that madness makes the sufferer unaware of what they are doing. Their positive reaction is a little unrealistic as it is too considerate although Tragedy is not at fault as its function is to induce pathos rather than to be realistic.

Euripides is the pioneer for psychoanalysts such as Freud and Jacques Lacan. Imagine a sufferer of bipolar effective disorder believing that they had discovered time travel during an episode of mania. This view would make complete sense to the person in

---

[32] Bennett in his book "MAM" neglects to mention this point and this critic views that his failure to recognise this point is why he misinterprets Ajax stating that it is the most visual play. For the most visual play cannot neglect what is the most powerful moment (coming out of madness) and what would also be a most visual moment.

this manic state. The Maenads in the Bacchae experience the same elation. When the sanity of the time traveller or Maenads is restored both realise that their behaviour was in a way possessed. The person has a chemical condition whereas the characters are forced into their behaviour because of a god. Both conditions of elation are not worth it in the end, for the coming out of madness is a considerably worse experience. This explains the most important phenomenon of the madman which Greek Tragedy presents in a frightfully realistic, chilling and gripping manner.

Please Note:

Any conclusions I reached during my dissertation on what constitutes Madness where views I had at that particular time. For example, I now know that there is no truth about madness being a chemical imbalance in the brain and psychiatry is at worst a complete lie and at best a metaphor. I know that we can alter our chemical state by changing our physiology. In 1998 I was not completely aware of these facts.

CHAPTER 3

BREAKING THROUGH

Breaking Through records selected thoughts after A Can of Madness was published. It started as a sequel then I realised that I was doing more good by helping people who came in to contact with me so I focused on growing Chipmunkapublishing more than on my own writing. I have chosen to include it extracts from it in 'Curing Madness' so people can understand how Chipmunkapublishing evolved after A Can of Madness and how improved my well being and continued to develop my own creativity. I also wanted to include how I came off Efexor as this was the first step to coming off psychiatric medication for good.

i) Punching through the wall

I was a raver that had a bad time... Such a bad time I didn't do much raving. But I lived and breathed it from the age of fifteen to seventeen, 24/7. There really were 20,000 hardcore knocking at my door. I could see them. It takes time to recover from taking five billion ecstasy tablets... one for everyone in the world... and then setting up a European Hardcore Committee, and heading it to instil world peace... that took a lot of effort... It was also a lot of responsibility...

I had to make sure that every girl in the world knew what it was like to be made love to... That was the best bit, and all it took was a bit of concentration, a bit of imagination you might say... It was a great feeling to make so many women happy... Then that in turn made their men... and other men happy (joke).

Follows naturally I suppose... Oh, but then I realised I was God... or was it Jesus. That was when it became too much to handle... It was too great a responsibility... I immediately felt guilty for all the pain and suffering in the world... Had I caused it? If I was omnipotent why couldn't I prevent it? Something had to be going on... Something underhand... Something dirty... Something sinister... and I was going to do something about it... Nobody else was doing it... Nobody else was capable...

Well something was going on and the media and the status quo have always feared it. There is a huge amount of stigma and discrimination attached to it across the board. That is why people who have "mental health issues" are commonly believed to breakdown, and not breakthrough. Well if that's so, and they are right, then I have broken down four times and not broken through yet. I mean, being given the label of someone who has bipolar effective disorder - no wonder I am programmed to think that I will always be liable to breaking down and that I can never be repaired, only at best patched up. Like a beaver dragging a tree across to a leaking dam, it seems impossible when you first see it. How do people recover from going loopy like that?

Breaking through wasn't even meant to be in my vocabulary. So when I broke through, as I call it, I was delighted. Delighted for myself because I had been through one hell of a ride, and delighted for others who had faced similar circumstances. Through what I had done I was able to create a platform for others to shine.

Other people who just needed an opportunity to be given an Equal life, whereas previously they had never had an opportunity so I set up Equal Lives. See www.equallives.org. Well, this was my mission; to create a movement that the likes of men like Nelson Mandela or Gandhi fought for. Whenever we think of people like that, no matter how much money we have, no matter who we are, we all feel humble. That is the essence of humanity for me. We are all so weak and yet so strong and that is what pulls us together as well as pushes us apart.

So why was it such a fight for me to get my first book 'A Can of Madness' in the public domain? There are several reasons. Having a manic marketing it i.e. myself was one difficulty, who knows, maybe it helped. Well that is because manic depression is a taboo subject; people don't want to talk about it, even though mental health affects all of us in some way. After all, we all have it.

We all have mood swings and we are all influenced by circumstances and day to day activity. Some of us more than others, that's true. Some of us can hide it away, some of us have better coping strategies but we're all human. That is what makes life exciting, what makes life durable. Without pain and pleasure it would be monotonous and two-dimensional. None of us can deny that we are vulnerable and this is how I chose to define the term mental illness.

In April 2002 I had the book launch for 'A Can of Madness' in the Lavender pub in Vauxhall. This would start me on a tiring journey in which I would commit to making the world a better place to live in for anyone who had been discriminated against, primarily mental health service users. Little was I to know what was to lie ahead.

It was the relentless manic energy that kept me going, that and the feeling that I knew what I was doing was essentially good for people who had been through a hard time. I never intended to be moralistic, or too pushy, in your face even, just believed in the concepts that I had created and wanted to develop them so that I could help every future manic-depressive in the world. Then, if I could help a manic, I could help a schizophrenic. If I could help a schizophrenic, I could help the homeless, drug addicts, ethnic minorities, the disadvantaged. I could change the establishment. I knew I would have to form alliances and I was prepared to sacrifice my life and privacy to just have a glimpse of a chance of changing the world in a small way. This was all possible, that was just about the only decent thing I learnt from the futility of Bacchanal raving. "Do what you want to do" was the old hardcore adage. So I did what I wanted to do. I mean, who doesn't, but things weren't easy, there was a lot going on.

I had to put up with other people's agendas, that was a difficult thing to come to terms with in the charity sector, especially when people are at first so friendly. It took me a while to come to terms with this. It's very hard to get a foot up. I'd self-published my initial book on the back of a Mind Millennium Award and distributed it to 300 charities and groups across the UK.

I'd met a printer on the way, Andrew Latchford, who encouraged me to set up a publishing company. Why not? I had no other form of income and we could sell my book through the company. So in August 2001 at the Mind annual conference I went round telling everyone about a website that never existed and a book that had not been finished. Fifteen months later I would be returning to do a book signing and waving a hand puppet Chipmunk around, who I was throwing around the stage. Why? Well my life had changed somewhat I guess.

Before I dive deeper into the mental health movement and my role within it and outside it, as an author, self-publicist, activist, speaker, politician, charity director, entrepreneur and public figure, I have a message for any young people who come close to losing their sanity. I hope enough young people will read this book and other positive stories written by people who have been mentally ill and that these books will make a difference, as it is the young generation of today who will have the power. They will be capable of reducing stereotypes and discrimination and change the media's negative attitude towards people with mental health issues after I'm gone.

It is young people who will shape the world in the future. At 30 I can still do a lot but I am already working with young people with The Chipmunka Foundation to encourage them to take over issues that the status quo cannot.

I shall begin by delivering this message in potentially the most powerful art form to do good in the next one hundred years. Rap music in my view, if it blossoms, will incorporate the ideals and dreams of the British youth. Let's face it, we're never going to have everyone going to the opera and listening large to Beethoven and Mozart. That is not to say that the amazingly peaceful and "traditional", aristocratic end of music can't be made more accessible, it can. Just read the rap and imagine it being played out to you by someone who cares about society, a philosopher even.

I'm writing a 100 raps to recovery
What the hell is this?
Yes .....
It's some kind of discovery
To raise awareness on mental health
And give us all some kind of real wealth
That is in your soul and not just your bank
account
Because it's time to surmise,
Surprise and work out an account
Of how far you are prepared to go
To let all of the brothers know
What life is like inside the mind of a madman

Gonna stay pro-active and listen to the sad man
Was that s a a ad man or s A A D HA M M
Getting political now cause that's one way to go
If you wanna change the world then go with me
flow
Before other people die and the flowers they
don't grow

I'm looking into implementing regeneration
in Lambeth, that's for Equal Lives
Gonna sort out my own borough, then do one at
a time
Want to help Southwark out but they are doing
real well
And my head starts spinning and my mind's in
hell

Cause if I see too much suffering I'll be back in
the bin
Like being dropped by vintage Mike Tyson and landed
on the chin

The rap above shows how difficult it is to help others when you are struggling yourself. What's needed is pro-activity, strategic planning, a good heart and good people amongst other things. For some it is too late, but they too still inspire and can leave their legacies.

Starting my second 100 rap to recovery on
Christmas Eve
I've got many pieces of armoury hidden in me
sleeve
Too late for Pete Shaugnessey I do believe
(Respect – Respect to this man – he did
what very few others can)
An inspirational super user who helped people
breathe
Gonna gain more momentum now that he has
gone
May the force be with me like Luke Skywalker
and OB1
Madpride and A Can of Madness they are one
of a kind
Neither of them is afraid to speak their own mind
Gonna save the user movement at the end of the
day
All of these individuals belong to us survivors in
some way
Now I've made my point I hope I can hear you
asking
How can I really help instead of multi tasking?

First you must make sure you can look after
yourself
It's unfair to bring your burdens onto someone
else's shelf
When your mind is steady and you're ready for
action
Send me an email and we'll start the contractions
Breathe in for Chipmunkapublishing and out for
Equal Lives
These are both my creative visions, a limited
company and a social enterprise
Chipmunka publishes the stories of the mentally
insane
Equal Lives helps the poor communities who've
suffered similar pain
Both give the opportunity to live a better life than
before
So there's still hope for you if you listened to too
much hardcore
So if you see a rap event in your local
neighbourhood
Look out for the =Lives sign and motto we're
doing some good
Like Chipmunkapublishing we are saving lives
Take the positive out of the negative and
compromise.

Raps like these can be versed or adjusted to a
global scale but then they are more likely to be
misinterpreted. It is a dangerous tool that can so easily
lead to gang violence and shootings and chasing the
American Dream. Just as stories like 'A Beautiful Mind'
can be fictionalised because they have to adhere to
Hollywood Liberalism. My wish is for this not to happen
to 'A Can of Madness' or any future dramatisation of a
story on manic depression that is written in the same

vain. That is why I want other people to make films of it. There are different versions already in the pipeline. I found the first interpretation hilarious, as it was so different to what actually happened and seemed so absurd.

All bodes well for the future… I think… Yes… Two Oscars… One for best screenwriter and one for best director of 'A Can of Madness'… both in 2007… no that's too soon…2010… I'll be too old by then… and I'm more ambitious than that… let's settle for best screenplay in 2007… ok…ok…

Whenever I used to tell people this, they thought I was crackers. So I tend to hang around with a peer group with higher standards to confirm my self belief system.

Well, some people would look at my medical history and think I'm crackers anyway, so what's the difference. I've been a certified nutter for twelve years. Nothing has changed now, not in the eyes of the status quo, society, I've just told everyone about it that's all. Something changed for me though… and this is what gave me will power to go for my dreams. My philosophical view on madness developed after all the psychoanalysing I went through in my first book.

At the end of 'A Can of Madness' I was grateful for the cognitive therapy I'd gone through, grateful I was still alive but had no real philosophical depth on what I had experienced. I was simply too close to the abyss.

My major concern was to go around the country defending what I had written to people who might not like the book. I knew the memoir would upset my family. My grandmother tore it up. I knew it would upset my friends. I nearly fell out with one of the best friends I could ever imagine, let alone had and still fortunately have. I knew I would offend some women with my previous "misogynistic" antics. I knew the language would put a lot of people off but at the end of the day I'd prepared myself for all of this before. I was ready for it and have faced and will continue to face. As far as I am concerned people can like or dislike the book but to assassinate me as a person or the syntax of the book is a little unfair. That wasn't the point. The point was to reach out to others who had gone, and will go, through what I went through. Re-writing it was like reliving it. By the time I'd finished writing it I couldn't keep rereading it. I was still in shock.

I thought it was going to be a national success the day it came out. Rather like those manic moments... Sometimes positive feelings surfaced but always with the intense paranoia behind them. I was unable to determine what was really going on. I mean I was labelled with manic depression at 17 and had been on drugs before. I didn't know what being normal was like.

At the time of writing this I've swapped my anti depressants around. This was 6 days ago. Now I have 150mg of Venlafaxine in the morning instead of at night. This means I am less high and more real. More normal and more tired... More focused but less energetic... More focused and more set in the real world... but, after all, what is real? I wouldn't know what real was now if it stood in front of me and slapped me in the face. I'm also on a mood stabiliser – Sodium Valporate and an anti psychotic – Quetiapine. The

Venlafaxine brought me out of my last depression. It helped save my life, or was it really me that saved my life because many people commit suicide when on and when trying to come off this terrible drug. I feel that somehow I am being lied to and psychiatry is the world's biggest propaganda tool. The drug companies use the psychiatrists as their drug pushers. Maybe I was lucky that I met a nice one or maybe I just had the luck of the draw or even the mental tenacity not to throw in the towel, yes like Rocky Balboa.

I've never tried committing suicide but I've spent two years of my mood well ingrained in the suicide mindset. It was only a few weeks ago that I first came up with a way of explaining how my friend felt when he committed suicide.

After a month's break I decided to carry on, with this that is. *Me moods been a bit up and down me lads and lasses. The transition from taking the Venlafaxine at night to in the morning is pretty mind blowing to say the least.* It's almost impossible to explain to a doctor or anyone for that matter. Also, a couple of times I've taken the pills at night instead of the morning, missed a dose, as if you take too much you go high, and then resumed. So I'm on the edge somewhat.

It was my birthday yesterday, 28, 21st of February 2003. A Pisces on his way to Hollywood who dreamed that coffee and cream at the Ritz costs £175. I went to where the cash register was and saw an old man with glasses sat down as if he was typing. This was reminiscent of my friend John Calder, who published Samuel Becket's poetry in the nineteen sixties. At one time Calder had 18 Nobel Prize winners on his books. Now he is struggling with the modern ways of the electronic publishing and printing world. He has an intellectual reputation that is well respected however. I gave a talk at his bookshop in Waterloo in January 2003 and the place was packed. Sixty people plus – it got a mention in the Guardian, which was my first mention in a national broadsheet as far as I am aware.

Then a few weeks later I appeared with my girlfriend Sonia in the Telegraph. I was the subject of a feature in the money section. This article was to have a massive impact on my life, but not due to the publicity that went with it.

Someone had seen the article in the paper that stated I'd sold 2000 copies of A Can of Madness. The same person had seen the fact that I received money from housing benefit and Income support as well. Then they sent the article to the investigator's desk. I decided to make plans to escape from the benefit entrapment by the first of April. I refused to get lost in the negativity that the benefit system engulfs you in and within 6 weeks had broken out of the system and taken the bold step to grow my mental health utopian mission and look to manufacture a way of providing employment and self value to anyone who has ever been diagnosed with a mental health issue.

The article forced me to reassess my life and make changes. The experience had a positive outcome as it resulted in my decision to commit 100% to my mission to change the way the world thinks about mental health. Advice for service users and employment, DLA, advocacy etc... The information reported in the article was false but forced me to get out of the benefits system which turned out to be a step forward.

Meanwhile Jamie, a fellow manic I'd met in a coffee shop in Green Park in February 2003, had done my first portrait. It inspired me to publish my third rap to recovery which I started to write in his presence.

I'm looking at the picture and it's got to be said
This guy is a manic he looks off his head
Yet controlled in some way me thinks as well
Keep rapping and drawing like this we'll be doing swell
Against the odds and we're one of a kind
The start of equality for the mentally ill I hope you find
Like gay people started to be accepted when I was growing up
I turned to drink as an unaccepted manic but kept from throwing up
Felt so much pain that I made my stomach so strong
On the outskirts was tough on the inside was wrong
Took years to accept it then I got right
Determined to spend the rest of my life making a fight
For the rights of the mentally insane
Whatever happens it will not be in vain
There's a connection with us manics like a parallel universe
The status quo is scared so it places a curse
But anything that's misunderstood is treated this way
Rise up to the challenge and win the day

Educate the media and public and fight for
Equal Lives
We'll go Gandhi way before we use knives
How will we they treat us in 50 years time
Will they be embarrassed to be a friend of
mine?
We're all human at the end of the day
A slight change in psychology then we've made
our point
People will have empathy no need to smoke a
joint
Eliminating psychiatry with the help of
psychiatry itself
An ideal to strive for to contribute to our mental
wealth
Our mental health is getting better every single
day
I hope to share this with millions of people
When we have the mental health live aid one
day
This will be my first global rap performance in
public live
I'm a buzzing messenger from the mental
health hive
You try to get rid of us we'll sting you back
We fight for equality from the average hacks
Too many people and faces are fighting
together
A community growing forever and ever

I found I could only write a part of the rap in
front of Jamie. The experience of having the portrait
being done was absorbing my mind too much. This
though was a pleasant experience as my passion for
my mission is so strong that it is only on rare occasions
that I can lose my head in the creativity of others. This

is something I strive to do all of the time but something that I find so difficult. It is as if the artist within me is always manoeuvring itself to be out in the open. Without being on the surface it would suffocate and I would die.

The need for a creative outlet is something that is necessary for manic-depressives. This is why I set up Chipmunkapublishing as "The Mental Health Survivor's Publisher". Writing helped me to express myself in ways that I would be unable to otherwise. It gave me a voice in the status quo where otherwise I would be silent. Without these words writing them, rereading them and uttering these words my mouth would be dry and my sight would be gone. I would be unable to smell the part of the human spirit that makes me want to be a part of mankind. I would not have wanted to rejoin society, certainly not in a positive or meaningful way.

So writing has been more than therapy for me. It has released the pain that I had and helped construct new belief systems that I have. It has saved my life. The more and more I realised that writing helped me and the more I realised that it would help other people I came into contact with in the mental health movement. The writing of my book became a symbol of freedom from oppression in the way that people with a mental illness suffered from stigma and discrimination. The more I delved into the unjust world of mental health politics and assimilated it to my own view of the world and how the mentally ill were treated, the more my life became a mission to help others the way that I had somehow managed to help myself. This mission was a humanitarian one and remains so. It's born out of human instinct.

On October 19th 2002, Chipmunkapublishing released its second author Dolly Sen, and her autobiography The World Is Full of Laughter. I'd met Dolly a few months before when we were both helping mental health user groups in Lambeth. We swapped email addresses and away we went. Dolly is very shy in person and extremely active. She is one of the most charitable and selfless people that I have ever met, always helping people who are worse off than her.

Reading my book encouraged Dolly to write her own story. When I first read it I had a tear on my cheek for half an hour. The fact that my story could have inspired someone else gave me more strength to carry on the fight for justice. Through reading the book it was clear that Dolly had gone through the same cathartic process as I had. In her own amazing words "This book started out as a suicide note and ended up as a celebration of life". Dolly has had thirty years experience working as an actress and she refocused me on my dream to take my story to Hollywood and write it and direct it… how it really happened.

ii) Dolly Sen

I never aspired to be a publisher. I never even intended to write a book, especially an autobiography. I knew I would write a screenplay and had planned to be a film director but somehow I had allowed myself to get side tracked into doing this. It was for a great cause though and it was worth it, to help people like this. No-one else would help them get their books published. It was not financially viable for mainstream publishing companies to publish stories of mental distress. People do not want to hear depressing things. People run away from pain and the truth in this regard. It is a natural human instinct to protect oneself from this kind of unnecessary pain. Life is difficult enough to handle as it is.

As my confidence was growing I realised that I needed more from life than publishing. I needed my own importance to be recognised in a direct manner. I had a craving for fame. I wanted to use the celebrity status that I was going to achieve for the social good. Anyone who didn't believe that this was going to happen I would eject from my life. It was time to surround myself by only positive people.

People who believed that my dreams would come to the foreground and become an integral part of my life, as I lived them out. There was no reason that I could not fulfil all my other intentions, as a rap superstar, Oscar winning screenwriter and Hollywood film director whilst expanding Chipmunkapublishing and developing the Chipmunka Group. Confidence was the key, networking in the right circles and enhancing my delegation skills.

During 2002 I had promoted my story A Can of Madness. January 2003 until June 2003 had all been about planning. Redesigning www.chipmunkapublishing.com and developing a business plan with the Department of Trade and Industry. These strategic steps would ensure that Chipmunkapublishing would have a future in the 22nd Century. This would be a legacy that would have recorded a new genre of mad literature. It was a long-term plan to protect the social evolution that was taking place. The madman and/or woman would be accepted in society and would once again be revered instead of feared or ridiculed at every opportunity, by members of the status quo.

During the first six months of 2003 I also worked very closely with a man by the name of David Hart. A truly remarkable man with amazing energy despite having terminal cancer. He was a springboard for ideas and inspiration and a founder member of Equal Lives along with Dolly Sen. At the age of 64 David was Jewish and had a history as publisher of yachting and food magazines. He also said how he was a Times journalist for 30 years and was always taken to lunch by Rupert Murdoch every time Rupert visited London. I seized this opportunity and we became good friends. Once I'd read 'No Logo' I became more in tune with his Liberal principles and was really effected by what I'd read about Globalisation. What particularly upset me was the slave labour that all the multinational companies like Nike would impinge on its workforce. Once things got hot they would just move country and exploit another workforce. These companies would pay only a few pence an hour, with forced overtime, living at work. These were the victims of Capitalist society.

In September 2003 I'd gone to Sri Lanka for two weeks and it was the first time that I had witnessed poverty that was so widespread. It humbled me. It made me realise that mental health was only a drop in the ocean. I realised and registered that most of the world and the third world didn't even have the right to have a mental health problem. They had to worry about disease and starvation and civil war. It made me feel less sorry for myself and with hindsight made me realise that there was more work ahead for me to find like minded people, and find a solution for these issues as well but first I had to come off the medication once and for all. I mean I could not go about curing people if I hadn't fully cured myself.

---

iii) GOODBYE EFEXOR

This extract was written whilst I was coming off Efexor. This is a dangerous drug to come off I have heard of many people who have committed suicide as a result of coming off this drug. I have mixed feelings about it as when I went on it I was suicidal and within 4 weeks of taking it my suicidal thoughts have gone. Robbie Williams admitted he was hooked on this drug in a Daily Mail article in 2003.

This section entitled Goodbye Efexor is not meant to offend anyone. I have to publish it to describe exactly how I felt when I as suffering the severe side effects from coming off it. People should not be given medication as a first and only option. People are brainwashed into taking psychiatric drugs as the only option when alternative therapies and techniques such as NLP can have massive benefits and provide far better results. We should have the right to live in a world which doesn't focus on drugs as the solution when they are often the problem. Since coming off psychiatric medication myself in 2004 I have never been happier or healthier. This is a fact. Ask anyone who knows me personally. The people I condemn in this chapter are some of the most inspirational people that I know. This shows how devastating the side effects were, even though the drug possibly initially saved my life.

Fuck Robbie Williams, still hooked on that Efexor. A manic depressive I hear and he does not have the balls to come out and say that he's got it. Think of all the fucking good he could do if this was true and he did what I was doing.

I've just come off that shite, Efexor. Fuck David Beckham and his first day wearing a Real Madrid jersey. Fuck Gerri Halliwell and her two autobiographies in eighteen months. Fuck Celebrity. Fuck the world and its capitalist mentality. Fuck the way it discriminates and ignores the people who need the help. Fuck the developed world for holding the third world back. Fuck you for reading this and not buying it and fuck me for writing it and for feeling sorry for myself.

Twenty-eight years of age and writing my second autobiography which is going to be published on the 10th of October 2003. Fuck that day when it comes. World Mental Fucking Health Day. We've got a big spread in the Big Issue on that day, Chipmunkapublishing that is. That's the little publishing company I set up to empower mental health survivors and their carers. Fuck the company and fuck Andrew Latchford the guy who encouraged me to set it up. Fuck all the authors who contact me and think that I am going to make them all famous. Fuck everyone who contacts me and wants me to advise them on this that and the other. Fuck John Bird the guy who set up the Big Issue who stood me up in Baker Street last week and left no apology. Fuck all those charities who ask me to give talks for free and ask me to write articles for their shitty newsletters.

Fuck all those charities that manipulated me in 2002 and used me for their own PR and self esteem.

Fuck all the junk mail I have to open everyday from charities wanting another piece of me. Fuck everyone in the world for trying to prevent my insight and my vision coming through. Fuck David Hart from the Lambeth Strategic Initiative who acted as a mentor and spent five months still not paying the £1000 his organisation owed me.

Fuck my brother who owes me £1000 and has no intention of paying me back. Fuck him again for always asking me to give him more money whenever I speak to him. Fuck him for criticising the rest of the family. Fuck my mum and dad for not offering to assist with the fucking mortgage I am taking out. Fuck them both for remarrying and neglecting me and my brother. Fuck my step mum for "telling me that I ruined my life" the last time I was in Gloucester. Fuck my step dad for having cancer, still being alive and not letting my mum leave him and run off with her boyfriend. Fuck these drugs for making me think that I am gay.

Fuck the English fucking weather and fuck London for being up its own arse. Fuck the people in the city in their flash suits and cars. Fuck everyone who uses the tube and never makes any eye contact with me when I try and cheer people up. Fuck the British people for being so crap at foreign languages. Fuck the British music industry for being so simple and fake.
4th of June 2003

This is my life and these are my words. Nobody has altered them prior to publication.

The Efexor has now left my system. Comic Relief are playing football in the park. For the first time I notice the "All Nations Centre Apostolic Church" above me. An odd looking character walks by. I manage to turn my heart before him before he goes down St. Oswalds place. I stop on the corner of Wickham Street where Sonia got mugged. The guy who used to collect the glasses out in the stripper bar ignores me as I raise my eyebrows and write. He looks behind himself with guilt knowing I know something he doesn't know.

Coming off Efexor has been a blessing in disguise so far. I came off it immediately. I'd been going high so stopped the 150mg dose and then stayed off. My world changed as I came off the drug. I'd had a meeting with my caring Doctor, Teif Davies and my girlfriend. I made a conscious decision to come off it in a positive way. I thought of Dawn Rider and his anti drugs member's community in the US. They had sent me 54 case studies of people who had come off Efexor and committed suicide. I knew of the horror stories but I came off the drug in a positive light and this made me avoid any kind of cold turkey.

June 2003 was to be another turning point in the life of Jason Pegler. My computer crashed at the beginning of the month, a few days later I was off the Efexor. I was disorientated and confused. The computer crashing woke me up to the fact that I had been spending far too much time at home on the computer. I was turning into an introvert when what I needed was to see interact with society.

I set about seeing London via the buses. Gone were the days when I was going to rush around everywhere on the tube. I was going to take the bus and watch the world go instead of constantly trying to confirm my position.

My whole work schedule would change. Gone were the days when I would invite people round to Chipmunka headquarters for a meeting. I would observe London and see the key people. I would only speak to MD's and chief Executives when it came to sponsorship. Speak to people who made the decisions. Enough of this being polite and not getting anywhere like.

I'd decided that I was not going to be exploited by any of these charities anymore. Throughout 2003 every charity I'd met had tried to take advantage of me in some way or other and so had every business man. Well now the real Jason Pegler was arriving back on earth after suffering the side effects from this strong medication it was payback time.

I set about playing the game in my terms and on my own rules. June 2003 I went undercover, travelling around London, playing the fool, appearing on the outside as if I were a tourist. Asking people for directions when in reality I was directing myself. The more abstract things became, the more I understood them. Not because I was manic but because I had a sense of humour, I had my own vision and creativity and was not side tracked by the mission's and messages of others. I started to understand the world subliminally and in a practical way. I realised more and more that what goes around comes around. Jules Mascarenhas had taught me that. The Producer who made a documentary about me and two other depressives. Initially he had discussed 20% - 33% deal for me, and then when the filming was complete he offered me 1%. Well I signed it off and just requested 10 videos and the ownership of some photos he had taken for my book cover. I though that he had done those as a friend but had he hell. He was out to bleed me dry man, just like everyone else so it seemed, apart from people like Dolly.

Thing is, in life, you need to know when to let go. There is no point in wasting energy. Remember in the Bronx Tale when the boy is chasing the guy who owes him $30. His gangster mentor, Chaz Palminteri, comes over and says well done. You got this guy out of your life for thirty dollars. Leave it. "He's a bum". Well Jules Mascarenhas you are a bum too.

Another rule I learnt in June 2003 was to only deal with the facts. Lambeth Strategic Initiative had received a cheque on behalf of Equal Lives (the organisation I had set up to positive discriminate for people who do not have Equal Lives) on January 14th. Well after being told most days for five months my patience snapped and I had to demand the money back. The upsetting thing was that the co-chair of this organisation was David Hart, my friend, yet another mentor. The man I had based much of my social enterprise around since I'd met him in October 2002. After having a tip off from a couple of friends who made me question the genuineness of this man I became more aware and realised a big truth. One can only deal with facts in life and not on supposition.

During these few weeks I felt a huge sense of betrayal and confusion, especially whilst having the side effects of the meds. When I put the cheque into context it became more and more important. A man had promised me the earth and little, except handing books out he was meant to sell and giving me more and more responsibility for the community. I'd also been waiting for six months for an article to go in the Times. That just wasn't happening either. Things were starting to add up. It just went to show that you can't trust anyone in life except for yourself, not even your family and especially not single minded people running their own prjects. No wonder so many people have pets.

By the end of June 2003 I'd performed on stage with a short improvisation as a rap freestyler, MC JASE. My performance was at a Madpride event and had an audience of a hundred people. My confidence had grown and enthusiasm was sparked even more when I met this Rastafarian gent Fred Peters who set up Kennington Youth Club amidst the Brixton riots in the 80s. Fred played the piano as I rapped and gave me the confidence to improvise my rapping which I knew would take me on a fulfilling and empowering road where I could be a kind of Eminem, with a social meaning behind it.

iv) The significance of John Breeding

The moment I read John Breeding's book entitled "The Necessity of Madness" my perception of the "mentally ill" changed forever. I realise that mental health really is a social construct and something that the mind self manifests. I understood how psychiatry is a form of social control and that I could empower people so that they could make a full recovery. It was in the moment of my decisions that I decided to come off medication for good that I took ownership of my life again and became emotionally free of societies burden of living with manic depression.

Breeding made me really see that I could take those final steps to recovery and that if I combined his intellectual abilities with the coaching methods of Anthony Robbins that I too could change the world and make the world a better place. By consistently caring about the "mental health" of myself and therefore other people I could encourage generations of people to step up and raise their standards so that they would refuse to be "mentally paralyzed" by their own fears and the inadequacy of the status quo.

Just as Michael Moore so cunningly reveals the other side to Bill Clinton and the White House, I could focus on a positive image on "mental health" that would create the first brand of its kind.

Chapter Six

Raps to Recovery

Any lyrics written below are not meant to upset anyone or incite any kind of violence. The lyrics were written whilst I was on psychiatric drugs and were the beginning of the development of my style as a rap artist. Any reference to language that could be deemed offensive has been published to illustrate my feelings whilst experiencing side effects on various medications. I believe that rap music can be used as a means for freedom of expression and is therefore a force for social good.

The Jason Pegler Announcement –
Raps to recovery

Anyone trying to use the work of MC Jase will be crucified. Need I say you?! That includes you, Mr Mel Gibson, your father and Quentin Tarantino – unless you pay Jason Pegler 21/02/75 that's 21/02/75, 1 billion dollars up front and reduce world suicide you're at it.

MC JASE

I'm MC Jase
And I'm off my face
With my Mace
I'm a headcase
Certified as a nutter when I was 17 years old
Right now I've got hair no cancer so I'm not bold.
Enough to feel sorry for myself
This MC is always full of stealth
Leading an army empowering mental health
Taking time to build up my strength
Using different media types and length
Whole empire is growing by word of mouth
First North, West, East and finally South.
Too many tasks for the multi skilled
Keep observing others then get off those pills
3 months more of Quetiapine
3 years of Valporate then off the gin
Back to reality, human being again
Diary of a madman discriminatory like man.
Creative voice is heard in prose
Better than breaking somebody's nose.

3/4/01   Poll Vault

Here's a tune for vault recordings, you know who I mean.
I've been to fuckin' prison, at least, I might as well have been.
We're a hot new record label with lots of wicked stuff,
so if you've been listening to shit, we think you've had enough.
I've been rapping for a while, in lots of different ways.
Been through more shit than Eminem & I'm not afraid of gays.
I've seen a world of madness, where most people couldn't go,
and occasionally I return, when my mind goes to and fro.

I've got madness on the brain
(Cypress Hill thought they were insane)
and I know it causes pain,
But, I have to tell my homies,
'cause my thoughts drive me insane.

I saw violence growing up, in my home and neighbourhood.
I used to get badly picked on cause, my brain was fuckin' good.
There were NWA and 2 Live Crew for a teenager growing up
The only sense of security was my Alsatian pup.
There was petty crime and drug dealing that I undertook.
Sometimes I was rather fortunate to get off the hook.
There were women everywhere but not as many as Snoop,

and I've been so fucking sick; I'm still waiting for my coup.

I've got madness on the brain
and I know it causes pain.
But, I have to tell my homies,
to stop them from doing the same

I remember knocking out a copper, when my mate lived in a squat,
I was so fucking paranoid; I thought the place was hot.
When I told my teacher that I was dealing drugs at school,
she burst out crying and said that she felt like a fool.
I had a good education and didn't take advantage of it,
now I realise I was fortunate, and that I'd acted like a tit.
Never used to go to school, I would lie there in my bed.
If I had my time again, I know the books I would have read.

I've got madness on the brain (and it's driving me insane),
getting better at the game,
And I have to tell my homies,
to stop them from having the same.

Had so many fights, it's impossible to add them up,
won them all apart from one, but I never had a cup.
A sovereign ring broke my nose and I broke my jaw myself,
the scar on my face from a screwdriver arose from clumsy stealth.
So I've been through loads of agro and now I've quietened down,
and if you try to wind me up, I'll probably just frown.

Don't push me or my crew too far, cause you will never know,
how far we've come and been, and how far we're willing to go.

Seen madness now I'm tame (it was driving me insane),
getting better at the game.
And I have to tell my homies,
cause they've helped make MC Jase's fame.

When I operate on the mike, there are many things to do,
philosophise and educate, but mostly, I entertain all of you.
There were bad things in my early days,
but now I've changed my ways.
Now I'm a real citizen,
as the past becomes a haze.
Still mentally insane, and it's a shame, I'm not to blame.
'Cause it causes so much pain, to tell people my real name.
Must stay on medication, so I can rejoin my generation,
must not forget, or relapse, or I could embarrass the X.

I've seen madness; now I abstain (slow)
I've already made my claim.
I thank my homies, then and now,
for putting up with my burning flame.

Gotta get it right for the world,
make it all a better place.
And then it will be worthwhile, to have rapped.......
yours truly.......the lyricist........and MC Jase.

19/06/01   **Alcohol**

Things were going wrong when I used to hit the bottle
Used to sit there and talk about who I'd throttle
Now there's homies round these flats
And everywhere I go I'm surrounded by twats
But at least they know their hip hop
And I know I'm going to the top
Of the rap music industry
That's DJ Fraudster and me
The vauxhall boys gonna take over
A rapper and a composer
We don't give a fuck about no life
That's only covered in strife
Might as well just end it all now
Than try to figure out how
But then I guess that'd be copping out
And we're made of metal there's no doubt
We're gonna crucify the rest
Because together we're the best
Whether it's free style or rehearsed
Our magic bubble gonna burst
And we're grateful to Eminem
That mad rapper can be a gem
He's bringing hip hop over here
And that makes it really clear
That we're gonna go for it
Because we've been through too much shit
We're gonna bounce back off the mike
And mix some tunes that give a spike
Cause we're really into this game
And we really want and need that fame, MC Jase

Rhyme and Reason

Rhythm, rhyme and reason, is for all of the four
seasons
So when this rapper wants to show which route he's
gonna go
There's some logic in his mind and a story you will find
About the world.
Yeah the world and what it's like
About life; and all the strife.
About how to cope with it, instead of feeling shit
The troubles that begin
Whether big, fair, huge or thin
This rappers really gonna be
No 1 for eternity + philosophy
Cause I got poetry that makes sense
An understanding of anthropology that's intense
I gotta hold of the mike and I won't let go
Wanna make me famous and make some dough
So I can set myself up and my future family
(speed up) And prepare for any traumas that may
affect me
Gonna entertain the crowd in a different way
No bullshit, or gangster rap but memories from the day
Tunes that will stay in peoples minds
And words that are targeted to open blinds

Cause I want people to learn from doing wrong
And I want them to sing this song
I want their lives to be fulfilled
I don't preach, I'm just chilled

(Slow) out. That's child out.
And I've been there,
well into despair.

And I got out. Just about
and it was hard, to play my last card.
I kept guard and although my life was marred,
I escaped to have my music taped
And then a record deal,
hoes, nice suits and a flash car.

Vauxhall Crew

Rapping now for the Vauxhall generation
Dolly Sen's drum and bass, the new sensation
Council estates must get rid of crack
And get these broken community spirits back.
Time for the hardcore music to make sense at last
Things boring, normal, then too fast.
I'm just a manic depressive at the end of the day
Want me to get a job and join society, no way.
Too much stigma and discrimination going on round here
Feel guilty for mentioning it, must drink beer.
Something's not quite right me, rapping here today.
I'm white, manic, not homophobic or gay; at least that's what I say.
Social evolution is what's happening now
Multicultural society ends the racism row
Equal lives must unite across the universe
Positively helping the status quos perversed
I'm so tired now I could end my life
Preaching like a bell end about my strife
Mental illness is a horrible thing
Mentally ill in Amityville makes my ticker ringer
Laughing at reality is an ingenious way
To forget the fucking label that ruins my day
My friend jumped off a bridge not so long ago
Couldn't stop that but with these words I grow
Next time you see a schizophrenic in the paper
OPEN YOUR FUCKING MIND!
DON'T LEAVE THESE LUNATICS BEHIND!
Help them out
Cause we're all human beings at
The end of the day
Even us Manic Depressives
Who don't know what to SAY?

Time to heal

There's still time to heal. Time to heal, for real. Stop making bad motherfucka's and be more like brothers. So there's time to heal for real, and bad motherfucka's can turn into brothers. That's turn motherfucka's into brothers.

There's racism all over the world, so rap is everywhere.
Just listen to a great rapper, and tell me that you don't care.
They'll fill your mind full of truth, intensity, love and questions
That's with philosophy, psychology and their best intentions.

And in multicultural societies all over the globe,
rap is a language that can reach everyone's abode.
Get rid of the gangster rap lifestyle, that people aspire to,
and substitute it for real rapping, that makes people do what they do.

We can still keep the element of fun, shock and crazy shit,
but rid the world from images of nigga's causing all the shit.

Blacks have been oppressed and that's a fact,
time they made amends instead of getting whacked.
And if it takes a mad white man, to help them along their way,
Then so be it, I dedicate myself.
I don't care if people think I'm gay.
And I don't care if people think that I'm wasting my time
It's all mine and I'll do it without expecting a dime.

Because it's my craving out of a necessity,
want to help solve the disease I see,
People not together and fighting each other's ass,
when all they need to do is hut, hut, hut, look up and pass.

Yeah. Pass the ball to each other
And turn the bad mother fucker's into brothers.
Cause there's still time to heal.
Time to heal for real.
And I want to stop bad mother fuckers
and help turn them into brothers.
Then us brothers, can say thank you, to our mothers.

So next time you're burning some weed and listening to death row,
remember that if a brother pulls out a g-lock its time to go.
No need to hang around and act too tough,
Because one thing is for sure,
you've both already suffered enough.
Once you get away from the violence and killing,
can start enjoying things, and make life more fulfilling.
There are so many things, out there to do.
It's a tragedy to die young, a tragedy for you.
70% of rap records are bought by middle class whites,
so there's hope for the rest of us and room for more party invites.

Yeah. Pass the ball to each other
And turn the bad mother fucker's into brothers.
Cause there's still time to heal,
time to heal for real.
And I want to stop bad mother fuckers,
and help turn them into brothers.
Then us brothers, can say thank you, to our mothers.

As this rapper starts out his career,
there's one thing you should know.
He's gonna rhyme like kid n play and know exactly
when to let go
Of the mic to let the melody and backing vocals
intervene

Cause he has an intuitive understanding of narrating
the obscene
That's a comical element of rap that is always here to
stay
As there's nothing wrong with healthy sex not even if
you're gay
Better to have a world full of orgies and open sexuality
Than one based on vengeance
and shooting mother fuckers in the knee.

Juice and Gin

When you Dogg Pound Crew gonna let JCB come in?
I've spent all this time sipping on juice and Gin.
And I see the great Eminem,
so cool that he can't rap about race
Well I'm not afraid, 'cause I've been to every place.
Know what it's like to be mad, then you know what I mean.
I've endured it and recovered from it, you should have seen

SEEN IT.
Seen the shit.
And I've endured it.
And I've still got my wit

My heads going to explode 'cause I write raps so quick.
And I've got no boundaries, so I'm gonna make you sick.
And tell you of all the troubles in the world, that 2pac talks about.
And I'll be accurate as well, of that…there is no doubt.

About drugs, a life of crime (pause) bitches,
money and a life of irresponsibility (27)
About guns, sex, fighting, booze, prison,
and love, decisions and insecurity. (20)
There's nothing I won't tell.
I'll tell everything that's on my mind.
My honesty bodes well,
at least, that's what I hope you'll find.

Cause life's hit me so hard I've no longer got a guard.
I'm opening my heart for the benefit of art.

A music known as rap,
which upper class people think is crap.
But its music that is real,
that's music that you can feel.
Not like that ancient shit,
that makes me have a fit

Rap makes one feel at home...unlike the millennium dome.
It's more valuable than chrome.
Yes, more valuable than Rome

Rap is a kind of music that is here to stay.
Its essence is too important, for it to ever go away.
Compounding more out of racism in 60's America.
There are many scars that I'll be telling ya.
These mother fucka's ain't healed yet.
If you think they have, you're a fool, I'll bet.
Black people had a rough time at the hands of whites,
and their bound to want revenge from societies ugly shites.
Remember when a black man couldn't go in the same bar as a white,
well it takes a long time and a lot of education to forget that shite.

In time, generations can forgive that shit,
and rap is the only mass way to convey it bit by bit,
For church ain't that popular anymore,
it's too antiquated for the young.
They're more likely to get pissed off, get hold of a gun.
Get the bastards back for making them hooked on crack,
for if you move to the hood it's hard to get back on track.

There's a lot of discipline needed to make a good rapper,
need to educate, without preaching, and entertain the foot tapper.

JCB 1

Now ev-ery body <u>listen</u>… to me
Stepping up on this mike… is <u>JCB</u>
Joining my crew… is the thing to do
(That means) telling other people what happened to you
Honesty is the name of the game
Making other's feel the (empathy) for your pain.

It's time to take the ride that was slip – er, ey.
As Coolio did it, then so can we
No need for the gin we just need the juice
Cause Snoop Doggy Dogg is a bit different than Proust
He may (be the best) rapper that's still alive
But sometimes (that gangsta stuff stings) <u>like</u> a beehive

It can, encourage youngsters to get the wrong end of the stick
Make them sell crack and think through their dicks
Causing teenage pregnancy on the estates
Making life even harder than social policy dictates
Black people born into poverty all the time
Not surprising is it – really – that there's so much crime

I ran 100 miles to see NWA
Then the Fugees made me stop and find another way,
Developed my own philosophy to help the disadvantaged,
Reflected on my life – knew I was privileged,
2pac gave me strength to make my quest reality
Although he is dead he gives me psychic energy

Like O B 1 <u>Kenobie</u> in the (star wars trilogy)

let Darth-Vader <u>win</u> to deceive his enemy.
<u>Luke</u> felt the force and got stronger every day,
JCB will win YES I'm going to save the day!

Going to stomp all the crime by reducing ignorance,
First, bring different cultures together – give them all significance.
Lots of ways to do this – make them part of the UK,
join up with So Solid Crew – they may behave in a different way.
They describe things as they've seen them in Battersea they say,
so I give them my respect – now I should tell you about myself.

Born and bred in Gloucester with sex, drugs, booze, and women
Everything seemed stable until I developed manic depression.
Trying to stop a nuclear war that was only in my mind,
making all these assumptions that I could never find.
Went from mania to paranoia at the click of a manic gun,
I was certified a madman, therefore crazier than everyone.

When JCB was seventeen I was hospitalised for my mental health.
In the years to follow this would seriously affect my wealth.
Really hit rock bottom when I realised what I'd thought,
one minute saving the world then humiliated and distraught.
Spent six months mad and suicidal in a mental institution,

a miscarriage of justice planted the seeds for a revolution

Diagnosed with a mental illness it took ten years to accept it

I managed to sort my head out for the very first time...

Start bringing different cultures together and making them chime.

A Can of Madness

Now, I was forced to go into a mental asylum,
at seventeen years of age,
And some years later I wrote about it
and cried on every page.
It was not recalling the experience itself that made me
really weak,
but telling people about it and letting them here me
speak.

I spent a long time writing and getting my book
published.
The government gave me funding which stopped me
feeling dissed.
I would give the first 300 sales to charity,
Fuck me, thanks to mind,
I'd been given an opportunity.

There are so many things in life that I want to achieve.
But I only get so much time so it's difficult to
alleviate the pressure,
as I don't know where to prioritise
Cause I don't know about all that gangster shit,
I don't feel wise.

I grew up in Gloucester,
which I thought was really good
Cause there were so many nutters in my
neighbourhood.
Then one day I grew up and realised,
it was all an urban joke

Cause by the time I left, I'd kicked the fuck,
out of almost every bloke

Then I went to Manchester, to go to University
I was meant to study Classics but I tried to be a G.
With my mates working on the door, and me shifting my shit,
Life was made more fruitful with a regular piece of clit.

There were bitches and hoes more regular than before,
And it was nice to be called a stud,
instead of a fucking whore.
I was popular at Uni,
till my drinking took control.
I'd have six litres of strong cider,
then piss on the remote control

I was violent all the time, and generally depressed.
But when I played football I had the talent of George Best.
There were many things going on when we lived in Mosside.
Living next door to a borstal helped make us the law abide.

You see this started moral questions going on in my mind.
I became too drunk to do anything evil for mankind.
Recovery wouldn't happen for several years,
that's why my fucking memoir is so full of tears.

Jase August 8th 2001

Where is love

I was white now I'm black
In this multicultural trap
There's a vision of the world I have as well
To combat prejudice and stigma and remove this hell
A manic man, who's too scared to say it,
Once he reveals he'll have to pay for it

But the world is changing and societies gotta answer
Got me homies with me and my ghetto blaster
Doin' the right thing for the segregated
You are of the alienation that you've created
Accept people for what they are when you meet them
Don't judge pre-emp or abuse or try to defeat them

Where's the black representation in this society
Gangsta rappa's and priests only is not diversity
Everyone else come out of your shell
Let bygones by bygones we might as well.

Ode to Slim Shady

Eminem can fuck it
I'll saw his head off
and put it in a bucket

People call him the rabbit
That makes me Big Wig
god damn it
I can run 8 million miles
So watch it!
Hang on let me think
I can't saw an idol's head off
That would be very disconcerting.

Ode to Slim Shady 2

Been rappin 10 minutes,
Eminem can shit it.
Been a manic depressive since 17
and he thinks he's losing it.
Ain't got not grit for a bit, or a tit
I'm beat, I was neat,
but popped pills and was defeated.

Ode to Slim Shady 3

Eminem I want to love you
But my hearts not full of shit
There's people dying shady
And you joke in spite of it
My dad can't understand you
His wife thinks you're a Dog
I'm understanding what you mean
But you got to do it my way now shady.

8 Billion Miles

Another rap to recovery is stepping up tonight,
Regenerating the urban generation used to give me a fright,
Now it's an automatic humanitarian goal,
To take the community in and its heart and soul,
MC Jase alive returning to the house that Jack thought he built,
Too many mistakes in the box and they're covered in guilt,
Manufactured rappers not writing their own lyrics,
Feeling sorry for themselves their bullies and cynics,
Waiting for the sunlight to rise on this beautiful day,
Gonna stop this gangster rap nonsense and spread positivity my way,
Twenty four hours till things turn around,
Humanitarian goals for your breath, sight and sound,
Not born in the ghetto but been to hell and back,
Caused by ecstasy and a manic depressive attack,
Eight years after then I bounced back,
Cured myself and helped others to heal,
Thought I was crazy when I listened to Seal,
He's had his head together all this time,
With those mushrooms and strawberries,
Pink New Yorkers and awful hash coffees.
One street brawl lost and the next 50 won,
My life nearly ended before it begun,
Things going on, people too scared to face up to want their dream,
Receiving your destinies, easy, just don't let your brain steam,
Life is worth living don't ask me that question,
Stop using other models; make your own invention,
Equal lives for all and Chipmunks unite,
Publishing, media, film, internet and your fight,

To make things open up, door and front,
Smile, laugh, do a parachute jump.

Chapter Seven – Hello Hollywood.

In June 2003 I started filming for the very first time.

The Movie Script to "Cans of Madness" is a great example of an incantation[33]. When writing I imagined that the screenplay was already successful and that it had already reached Hollywood. As I now write we are already starting to make Chipmunka films in house. This comes across in the autobiographical script as well and was one of the main driving forces that enabled me to write it in the first place.

Another Incantation:

After 12 years of being on psychiatric medication Pegler I finally chose to come off the drugs with the help of life coach Anthony Robbins. By the time I finished this script I was nearing 30 and was Young Social Entrepreneur of the Year 2005. The crusade that had begun in 1993 at the age of 17 to break down the mental health taboo once and for all now had the ammunition it needed to deliver. All that is needed is to sell this script for an eight figure sum and produce films that will fill my utopian mission in house. Inside my heart is a mission to help other people, by changing the way Hollywood thinks about mental health and therefore, the whole world at large.

---

[33] Anyone who wants to learn more about incantations should read "Awaken the Giant Within" by Anthony Robbins.

Initial Cast Envisioned for:

A Can of Madness The Film

Jason – Jason Pegler/ Tom Cruise
Brad – Johnny Depp
Sonia – Penelope Cruz
Dad – Michael Caine
Harrv – Brad Pitt
Mum – Bridget Fonda
Gina – Halle Berry
Meredith – Nicole Kidman
Felix – Robbie Coltrane
Mark – Gary Oldman
Dom – Tom Cruise
Ed – Liam Neeson
Claire – Glenn Close

A Can of Madness

The Screenplay by Jason Pegler ™
December 2004 – April 2005

Part 1

Club scene: 5 min
Quiet Room/table tennis/changing clothes/brad leaves: 11 min
Internal dialogue 1 and 2/Prodigy: 5 min
Jason's Dad and Internal Dialogues: 7 min
3 months later: 1 min
Ward round: 4 min (33mins)

Part 2
Uni Fight scene: 4 min
Chorlton/moss/trav mania: internal dialogue. 12 min
Uni visit: 2 min
Dr Clarke's 3 min – Sunday coffee
Final exam tripping 5 minutes
Graduation =4m (+30m=63min)

Part 3
Prozac Nation: 5 minutes
Narrative: move to London, meeting Sonia, Miami 4 mins
Psychologist final Meeting: 3 meetings
Dr Davies meeting: 3 minutes
TV – 4 minutes
4 Writing and finishing script with Girlfriend 2 minutes
3 Making of film: 2 mins
2 Hollywood living + Oscars meeting Jack Nicholson/cameo role: 2 mins
1 Saturn and manic vision: 2 minutes.

The film begins in the depths of a hardcore club in Swindon in the mid 1990s. The atmosphere is dark, packed and extremely noisy with a 50K indoor system blasting out and an MC refusing to leave the stage. There are three people stood on platforms and the camera zooms in on one of them, a teenager called Jason. His eyes are dilated and he is sweating in a trance like state.

MC: 'It's ten past 3.00 in the morning and we're going nowhere. Speaker box climbers get off the stage you are distressing it for everyone. Now let's dance to some real deafening madness. Are you ready? That's nothing like loud enough. I said, are you ready?'

JASON: 'Can you dig it? Yes. I can dig it'.

MC Robbie Dee: 'I said it's gone ten past three in the morning and we're going absolutely nowhere. We were meant to finish at 3.00am but we are pumping up the hardcore especially for you. Right now...There is no escape... Loving it.... (Fantasia back to the future theme tune... lets go.... is here in the back ground...).

Jason starts matching the sound of the recorded tape in unison with the beat.

'Da da da da.. da da da... da da da da da da da...
'Da da da da.. da da da... da da da da da da da...

HARDCORE: Let's go... into the future

As the repetitive sounds continue Jason starts giving it the hardcore with all his might. He moves his whole body in time with the music and has an extraordinary amount of energy coming directly from his inner self.

He seems as though he is on some kind of spiritual journey as the deafening music makes 2000 people go absolutely mental. Back to the MC who starts shouting, interrupting the repetitive beats but somehow allowing them to continue and giving them new found meaning and enlightened significance.

MC ROBBIE DEE: (music from Fantasia Second Sight) To all of those who know the score how's about a little bit of hardcore... goes a little something like this... don't forget to hang the DJ... but not this DJ... for this is the one and only DJ Ratty... and if you double cross this DJ... there is only one way you can go... Straight to hell... dive into the abyss... and there is no way you are coming out. No way you're ever going to come out.... Because there'll be 20,000, yes 20,000 bleeding hardcore knocking at your door. No way out. Yes no way fucking out... so stay off those fucking speakers and pump up the hardcore...into the future...Into the future...Yes whaooooooaaayyy yeah (sound of woman's voice on tape), we'll live as one family.... Last one for the night for all you boys and girls here's MC Robbie Dee bringing it down... previously cooking up your brain... been cooking up your brain but now bringing you down softly.... Bringing you down nicely.... Alright matey.... Let yourselves go.....

Whaaaoooaaaaayy... whaaaoooaaayyy we'll live as one family..... We'll live as one family.........

This scene needs a lot of impact. It should be 5 minutes in length. (It could be a manic voice over or extract from the book about being a raver or manic moment epitomising excitement/narrow-mindedness/futility of rave culture).

The camera focuses back on Jason's forehead profusely sweating and onto his mouth singing the strong sounds of the woman's voice. Now into the mouth, and onto the next scene, where a tape is seen being played playing the same music from above.

Two young men, who look like ravers, are sat in an oversized room. They are in a mental institution. There are several old chairs and an old stereo. The curtains are open and it is dark outside. Noticeably there are great big bars on the only window.

BRAD: 'great night, I remember that one. That MC Robbie Dee is proper crazy. We'll live as one family. Wa ooohh yaaa. What did you say they call this? The quiet room hey... well its not the quiet room anymore... we've just impregnated it... Still I can see you need to get away from those loons in there and get some piece once in a while. I know I would if I were in here. How ya feeling?

JASON: Like I know the score... how's about a little bit of hardcore...

BRAD: You are still a bit off your head mate... how long you going to be in here do you reckon?

JASON: As long as it takes to save the world. I took 5 billion ecstasy tablets last night. One for everyone in the world, so I could create world peace by making the world live as one family. That meant that I could make love to every woman in the process. Not bad for one night's work.

BRAD: [Pauses looking worried for a split second] Wow really... don't worry mate you'll be out of here soon. You've got a good head on your shoulders. When you get better you'll be stronger for it. Your heart's in the right place.

JASON: Whhaaoo ayy. We'll live as one family. Want a game of table tennis?

BRAD: 'sure let's do it. Bro… let's go…

JASON: Into the future…

[A little pause, Brad looking worried, turns into a laugh and then a smile]

BRAD: You're amazing you are… come on…

JASON: Let's go… into the future…

[Brad laughs out loud]

They proceed into a white corridor and then into a big lounge where there are about 15 patients sat down watching TV. Most of them are smoking. A couple of old grannies are knitting. Coronation Street is on in the background. The game of table tennis is a strange affair. Both players are quite good being able to hit the ball over at a reasonable pace. Strange thing is that Jason tries smashing the ball when it does not seem possible. This must be a sign of boredom or perhaps he actually believes he can pull the majority of these ridiculously hard shots off. He tries ludicrous shots and loses the first game 21-11. Then just before the second game starts we start to get a real indication of just how off his head Jason really is.

JASON: I'm just going to change…Into the future. I'm going to get out of here now. I'll be back.

Jason walks backwards deliberately… pointing at his back while he leaves the room. Brad laughs and Jason walks out of the room, back towards the corridor where the bathroom is and along one door further down on the left hand side.

He goes into his room and puts on a hardcore tape (The producer and DJ Tanith – first 30 seconds Fantasia Castle Donnington). Jason takes his shoes off and puts on four pairs of socks putting his shoes back on. He takes his jumper off puts on a couple of T shirts and then a couple more jumpers, his puffer jacket, a woolly hat and another pair of baggy jeans. Finally he puts his gloves on and then goes back into the dining room. The table tennis table is away from the rest of the room. Brad manages to hide the fact that he is worried from Jason and joins in the manic fun.

BRAD: Are you warm enough Jase?

JASON: I'm freezing… I'm going to get out of here man. You know I stopped that nuclear war?

BRAD: That's good, shall we carry on playing?

JASON: Sure.

They play a coupe of shots where Jason tries ridiculous smashes.

JASON: I'll be back…

BRAD: I'll make a cup of tea. Do you want one?

JASON: ok…

As Jason leaves the room, the camera turns to Brad following him, walking out of the room along the corridor in the opposite direction. He looks more serious now, takes a deep breathe and looking a little worried puts the kettle on. He lights up a cigarette as he waits for the kettle to boil placing two mugs and making preparations for coffee. Jason comes back in dressed as he was before he put too many clothes on.

BRAD: You decided you were warm enough then.

JASON: Yes I'm fine now. I will get out of here though.

BRAD: I know you will Jase… I know you will. Here's your coffee. Don't pour it on your head buddy, remember. Drink it.

JASON: I like the taste. It will mean I can help more people, drinking this significant drink.

BRAD: [Looking a little worried] I see. So, when you going to get out of here then?

JASON: Some time soon. Some time soon.

BRAD: I'll have to go after this cuppa. Still knackered from weights and I've got work tomorrow.

JASON: I've got love making to do. So many women to see and men to stop from fighting. The world needs me. Now that I'm God and all, so much responsibility, but I enjoy it really you know Brad. I enjoy looking after everyone, especially when they don't know I'm looking after them.

BRAD: I know you do... [Rubs his eye] I know you do...

A big, fat, Welsh nurse called Gary walks in. He must weigh 20 stone, but looks kind. He looks at Jason.

GARY: All right Jase?

[He seems more interested in talking to Brad. They shake hands]

GARY: All right? Brad is it?

BRAD: Yes that's right.

GARY: You're a good mate you are. Come to see him a lot you do? I know Jason appreciates it you know. He lights up when you're here. It's important that he can see his friends.

BRAD: That's what friends are for. I'm sure Jase would do the same for me. Wouldn't you Jase?

JASON: Interesting coffee this. Very interesting. Can't remember how I stopped the nuclear war. How did I stop the nuclear war?

GARY: Don't know Jase. But somehow you managed to all right. There's not going to be a nuclear war anymore?

BRAD: That's for sure.

Gary and Brad laugh quietly.

JASON: Thank God... I mean, thank ME... God... for that...

Brad and Gary look blankly back at Jason. Jason does not pick up on their blank look.

JASON: Yes glad I stopped that. It wasn't easy to work out but I did well.

BRAD: Yes you did well Jase. You did well...

JASON: Thanks Brad. Thanks.

BRAD: We'll, I've got to be going now Jase. Duty calls. I've got work tomorrow.

GARY: Nice to see you again Brad. Come back anytime.

BRAD: We'll see you Jase.

JASON: I'll see you out Brad.

GARY: See you in a minute Jase. Don't be long.

BRAD: Well Jase, like I said, I'll see you tomorrow. You be all right? Make sure you don't run off. They're looking after you in here you know. I know it's hard, but you'll see.

JASE: Yes. But, I'm looking after them under cover, all of them and they don't realise it, but you and I know. Right? Promise me that you won't tell them? I have to stop the inevitable nuclear war again and make them understand.

BRAD: I know mate. I know.

JASE: Promise you won't tell them anything Brad, not until I give you the signal?

BRAD: You've got my word on that. I promise.

JASE: Safe.

BRAD: Safe.

They shake hands and Brad leaves the ward pushing his expensive mountain bike out. Jason looks like he may follow, when Gary calls him in the background.

GARY: All right Jase, come and play that game of table tennis now.

JASE: [Turning round] Yeah OK Gary. Going to have a cigarette and listen to some hardcore first though. I'm trying to crack some messages that the tapes are sending me, about stopping this nuclear war. See you in a minute.

Jason walks past Gary closes his door and takes out one of his Embassy Number one cigarettes.

(Internal dialogue 1 shows Jason in the exciting parts of mania)

JASON'S INTERNAL DIALOGUE 1: Nothing to do when you're locked in a vacancy. Now I see why John Hughes was telling Bender to stop that Nuclear War, but he didn't know how to do it. He didn't realise that it is the film director himself who does it, not the actor.

Like me, the film director of the world now. I'm filming everything that happens on earth as a movie through my mind. How clever. I'm God the ultimate Oscar Winner. It's so obvious. Can't believe I am the one, but I must be strong. People need me and most of them don't even realise it. Even those that do could never admit to it.

(Internal dialogue 2 shows the confusion and pain caused my mania and illustrate why it cannot be allowed to continue in the 'real world')

JASON'S INTERNAL DIALOGUE 2: Oh my God... that's me. So much responsibility and I seem to work out the answer... all the time... I work out the answers and it doesn't seem to make any sense... One minute I'm God... looking like Robin Hood. Next I've changed into the new Alex Ferguson or an abject slave performing rituals. What the hell is going on? I don't understand. So tired, my brain keeps working on over drive, yet it seems so automatic and I'm sure there is a cover up. Why are people trying to be my friends? Because they want to start the nuclear war... they want information from me... the chosen one... God... well I'm not giving it... I'm more cunning than they are... all of them... I won't give in... I don't take this job lightly... I haven't been going through all this to give it up to some conspiracy against the world... their creator... Gotta calm down and listen to this tape... the Prodigy will have the answer. Forget the Producer.

He plays Wind it up by the Prodigy. Jason starts to dance in his room like someone possessed in Brunel

Rooms in the 1990s i.e. like he was in the first scene but better and faster this time. When the first words of wind it up are echoed in the song the camera continues to focus on Jason dancing but the internal dialogue 1 comes back on.

Yes. Wind it up... Wind it up... I'm winding the world up... like an alarm clock... the world is in my hands... and I created to Prodigy to send this subliminal message to those in the dance world. I created ecstasy as a drug to create world peace and the singers and dancers to create harmony so that we do all live as one family. Then I needed to join the scene and release everyone's unconsciousness. Make them part of the real world. I started with ravers... then the rest of the world can unite and join together in perfect harmony...

Suddenly there is a knock on the door. It's Jason's dad.

DAD: Hi Jay. Can I come in? Do you mind turning the music down. I've brought you a couple of Mars Bars. Have you've eaten?

JASON: Yes, I've eaten thanks Dad.

DAD: Have one of these now then.

JASON: Thanks. I'm starving.

DAD: Must be those pills. You've put on some weight, but don't worry about that. We want you to get better first. And you needed to put on some weight anyway, I think. Did you sleep ok last night?

JASON: Yes thanks, I must have got seven hours sleep. Something like that anyway. Definitely got some sleep. Didn't think I was that tired.

DAD: That's probably the pills as well. They're bringing you back down. You have had so much energy for the last few months. Too much, in fact. It wasn't normal. Now you're starting to get back down to earth. It will take some time. Do you know what's been happening?

JASON: Not really.

DAD: The doctor has said that you have been high. Not in the real world. Manic he called it. Now they're giving you drugs to clear your thoughts. Make you what you were like before you got ill. I'm so pleased though. I thought you were a gonner at one point. I thought you were going to be a cabbage.

JASON: Why is that dad?

DAD: One day I came in and you didn't even recognise me. You were just that. Your eyes were like stone.

JASON: How did that happen Dad?

DAD: They had to restrain you. One day when I walked in you through a chair through a window and it took five nurses to bring you down. They had to put you in a straight jacket and injected you with some drugs to calm you down... (Eyes start watering)... It was really scary ...but it had to be done, you were out of control. Anyway the drugs they gave you were so strong that they knocked you for six. (Wipes tears from his eyes). And I thought you were a gonner, I really did. You know, I've got a friend with a son like you, who's been in a place like this. He said that his son's been sat there for two years. After two years he still doesn't recognise him.

JASON: That's sad dad.

DAD: Promise me you won't take those drugs again Jay. You've been really lucky, been given a second chance, you know? You have to take it.

JASON'S INTERNAL DIALOGUE 1: What about these drugs I'm taking now they're even better... ha hah haa and what's more, they're free and legal... As god I had to assume an antic disposition, but can't let this on, as I don't want to upset my dad now, or Hamlet or Shakespeare for that matter. It's a lot of responsibility being the father of God, so I better play dumb. Anyway I still take drugs, but only telepathically. They have more of an effect that way.

JASON'S INTERNAL DIALOGUE 2: But what if he's right. My dad. All these amazing thoughts I had. They can't be true. It's impossible and I could never admit that they were not true, that would be the most humiliating thing on earth. To admit to having lost my mind and to admit that I am actually living in a mental hospital. What a disaster. How can I ever look my teachers, friends, people I know in the eye ever again, without ever feeling like a loser, an animal even? How can I play Rugby again, go back to school, go to University and lead a normal and even an inspiring life, after I admit to having been completely insane? It's like Jack Nicholson in One Flew Over the Cuckoo's Nest, and it's my life. This is too much to bare man... no way... No way out of this mess... Ahhhhggghh....

JASON: I won't take them again dad.

DAD: Now you are getting better Jay, there is one thing you have to be prepared for.

JASON: What's that dad?

DAD: Well I spoke to the psychiatrist the other day and he told me that things are going to get worse before they get better.

JASON: Why's that?

DAD: Well he told me that now you are beginning to realise what has actually happened it's not going to be easy accepting everything and your mood will naturally go low.

JASON: What do you mean Dad?

DAD: Well Jay I mean that he said you're going to get depressed.

JASON: For how long?

DAD: Well we don't know exactly but it could be a long time. The important thing is that you keep taking the drugs they give you… I know you will anyway. What is also important, perhaps more important is that unlike a lot of the other patients in here you have a good support network. I mean a really good support network around you. You've got a good doctor. You've got me, your mum and your brother. You're Grandma and your Nan and you've got very good friends who come to see you Brad and Tim and Dom. They're all here for you. Have you seen Brad today?

JASON: Yes dad. He's been doing weights. Really strong now.

DAD: He's a really good friend you know. He comes to see you nearly every day doesn't he?

JASON: Yes dad.

DAD: You're a lucky chap. You remember that OK.

JASON: Will do.

Jason sparks up another cigarette and looks into the loving and distressed eyes of his father.

DAD: What did you have to eat for supper then Jay?

JASON: Fish and Chips and sponge pudding with custard.

DAD: When you come home we'll have Fish and Chips from Ready's. OK?

JASON: OK Dad. When will that be?

DAD: Don't know son. Won't be long. You just hang on in there ok.

JASON: OK Dad.

DAD: Well I'll be off then Jay. I've got work in the morning. Just wanted to say hello. Love you. [Kissing his son on the cheek and giving him a hug]

JASON: Love you too dad.

DAD: You'll be ok wont you. Just hang on in their kid. You've got the mental strength I know.

JASON: I'll see you out.

As they walk down the corridor the camera moves slower than usual.

3 months later in Jason's room. Jason is no longer manic. Over the last 3 months his mood has dropped. He has been in a suicidal state for a while and sleeping 16 hours a day. He has been given his own room still as his parents asked for him to have his own space. He is lucky in this regard as all the other patients are split in between two dormitories apart from another single room which is left empty for any pregnant women. He lies crying in his bed like a little five year old boy who has lost his parents when shopping at night and is afraid of the dark. Bob Dylan's 'Times Are Changin' is playing in the background.

Jason sits up and brushing away the floods of tears he picks up Nelson Mandela's autobiography 'Walking to Freedom'.

He cannot seem to concentrate so takes the book into the hall and sits cross legged in the doorway. Looking up as the day to day activity of the ward goes past. One of the nurses tells him to get up because it is medication time. He reads for a minute and then eventually keeps looking up. From where he is sat he can see the patients lining up and taking their medication one by one. A team of broken souls, longing for a better existence. If only Jason could put his own life in perspective with that of Nelson Mandela perhaps he would have a chance.

Quick flashback to 18th birthday in hospital: 30 seconds.

Fast forward 2 months and Jason is sat in a ward round.

DR.TAYLOR: How are you Jason?

JASON: A lot better thank you Doctor. I can't wait to go home.

DR.TAYLOR: We'll see about that. I have some questions to ask you OK. Please answer them as honestly as possible ok. I think you know the drill by now… Is life worth living? Yes or No?

JASON: Yes.

DR.TAYLOR: How do you feel compared to the last time I saw you?

JASON: I feel less depressed and more ready to go home.

DR.TAYLOR: Do you feel like you are likely to harm yourself?

JASON: No my mood is better. I don't feel suicidal now. I can see that there is light at the end of the tunnel.

DR.TAYLOR: So you still feel that you are in a tunnel.

JASON: No I feel like I have been in a tunnel and now I'm looking back. I have a long way to go but I'm definitely looking back. I promise.

DR.TAYLOR: Jason you don't have to prove yourself to me or anyone else here. You understand. You just have to be honest with yourself. I know it's difficult but you're doing well believe me. You've been with us quite a long time now. Six months I believe but there is a definite improvement OK?

JASON: Yes Doctor.

DR.TAYLOR: So you can see light at the end of the tunnel. On a mood of one to 10 with 1 being depressed and 10 being normal how do you feel?

JASON: Six I guess, maybe seven but that will go up to eight or nine if I can go home for good.

DR.TAYLOR: Do you have racy thoughts any more?

JASON: No Doctor.

DR.TAYLOR: Do you feel depressed?

JASON: I don't feel like I did before if that's what you mean. I mean I do feel depressed sometimes but I feel that that is because of everything that has happened and the fact that I am still living here. There's a lot to cope with bearing in mind everything that has happened. My life has been turned upside down.

DR.TAYLOR: I see. I believe you are seeing a counsellor Reginald every week. Tell me Jason how is that going.

JASON: It's going well. I like Reginald. We have some good talks. I can tell him things that I don't talk to other people about. Personal things you know and I can see its helping me deal with the situation, the past, the present and the future, in a way that I never thought possible, until I met him.

DR.TALOR: That's good Jason. How do you feel about other people?

JASON: What do you mean doctor?

DR.TAYLOR: Do you like them? Do you feel resentful to them in anyway, angry even?

JASON: No doctor, not at all. I feel embarrassed maybe, humiliated even, because of all those crazy thoughts I had that were I thought were true… thinking I was God and all that. Apart from that I just want to rejoin society and I'm ready to go.

DR.TAYLOR: Well I think you're nearly ready to go now Jason. You can go home this weekend and then I'll see you next week. Should you continue to improve and the medication continue to work, which there is no reason why it shouldn't I'll see you once more next Thursday and then you'll be ready to go for good.

JASON: Really Doctor, it's great. Thank you so much.

DR.TAYLOR: Well I think that just about wraps it up for today Jason if you will excuse me. Please can you ask Harry to come in?

Jason leaves the ward round for the first time ever with a smile on his face. He goes to the main lounge where there are several people watching TV and sees Harry biting his knuckles.

JASON: Harry you are next.

HARRY: What ward round Jase.

JASON: Yes Harry.

HARRY: You look happy Jase. Good news.

JASON: Yeah Harry. There going to let me go next week. Don't believe it.

HARRY: Well done Jase. Wish me luck hey.

JASON: Good luck Harry. Good luck mate...

HARRY: Can't remember where the door is Jase can you show me? I can't remember anything since I started this ECT?

JASON: Here it is mate. Here's the door. Allow me.

---

15 months later. September 1994. It's Jason's second year at Manchester University. He's watching match of the day drinking some cider in some run down house with a big TV when the door bell rings.

JASON: I'll get it its Meredith.

ROGER: All right Jase.

Jason opens the door and a pretty girl with blonde hair dressed in a short dress and lots of make up can barely speak. She's crying her eyes out. Jason lets her in.

JASON: Hey... what's wrong?

MEREDITH: Th... That bastard out there tried to kiss me and the only way I could get him to stop was by telling him that he could come back with me. When I answered the door he ran off.

JASON: You what... You fucking what... Wait here...

MEREDITH: Wait... come back.

Jason races out of the flat and Meredith stays in the hallway. Jason runs round the corner and sees the bloke walking away.

JASON: Oiiihhh. I said Oiiiihhh. You.

The man turns round in the dark. Jason can't see his face. Jason runs right up to him.

JASON: That's right you... you mother fucker.... Who the fuck do you think you are..... [punching him in the face he falls to the ground and Jason starts kicking him in the head repeatedly].... Who the fuck do you think you are... whack... fucking with my bitch like that... doosh... You like hassling women do you.... You fucking gutless turd...thwacckk.. You think your going to get away with this.... Kapppooww. You just picked the crazy person in Manchester to fuck with.... Smack. [Jason then kneels on top of the man and starts punching him in the forehead, eyes and nose. After about fifty punches he regains his breathe]... I was in the bin you know... and now I've got to put up with a prick like you.... Fucking with my girlfriend like that... she's done nothing. [Standing up and kicking him in the head a couple of times and on his back and arse]. If I ever see you in this neighbourhood again or hear from you ever again you're dead. Now get the fuck out of here or I'll kill you. You mother fucker.

As Jason walks away he can see Meredith watching in the back ground. He gives her a hug and they go back inside. Meredith goes upstairs to freshen up and Jason goes back in to watch match of the day.

JASON: I just kick fuck out of this bloke who was molesting Meredith.

ROGER: You should have said we'd have helped you mate.

CHRIS: Yeah. I thought I heard something. Is he still outside.

JASON: Don't know.

CHRIS: Let's have a look. I'll come with ya. For protection, not that you need any Jase.

They walk outside and there is no sign of the man. Jason goes down to the floor where he was on top of him. There is a pile of blood and then a trail going down the alley.

CHRIS: Looks like he got the message Jase. Don't think he'll ever come round here again. Gonna watch the rest of Match of the Day.

JASON: Yes.

CHRIS: Come on Manchester United are on next. I'll make Meredith a cuppa. You want a lager. I've got some. Tastes better than that crap you're drinking. Not so strong but tastes better for once. You might have got lucky. Could have got a Leeds fan there you know. Come on mate. Let's get back inside its cold out here.

----

12 months later there has been heavy drinking... stopped taking medication nine months previously... no symptoms of manic depression until...

JASON'S INTERNAL DIALOGUE 1:

Jason narrates with Meredith now openly Mistress Real, asleep living in a quieter area in Chorlton Cum Hardy. He begins believing Chorlton is the head of World Consciousness and the whole world is a brothel.

There is a visual re run of events. Talking is in the back ground. (Like the big fuck you scene in Spike Lee's 24 hours)

Ah what a privilege it is to live at the head of world consciousness and to be the first to realise that the whole world is actually a brothel. As I stand here an abject slave to the Mistress of the night. The camera zooms in on a picture of Mistress Real sat in her purple throne. She also happens to play the character of Meredith. The most intelligent Classics Professor of my tutors had an inkling no wonder he was bordering on the insane.

Not like me God aka Jason Pegler, an undercover Classics Student and manic depressive from Gloucester understands the real significance that I can indeed create world peace by forcing the whole world to make love to each other in a subliminal and a pro-active way. I will have to withstand pressure from all my sides from other Dominants and make my move now.

As I masturbate while looking through my window I can see a light on. Behind this light I can feel myself making love to the beautiful horny middle aged woman inside. As I awake her from her sleep she has multiple orgasms and starts to dress up in her leather gear placing a whip between her panty hose. The world thought that the sub dominant scene was something to be criticised for pain and humiliation. Well once everyone goes through the real physical pleasure and trust that stems from this movement even only in an unconscious level they will be nicer to their fellow man and start to give instead of taking. That includes giving more head… Ha ha Ha ha…

I look at my girlfriend while she is asleep. Mistress Real. She is so caring looking after my every need in the real world appearing to be my Mistress and this is what I must make her think. As I discover the ultimate sense of trust and faith from womankind through my relationship with her I can manipulate others and go through each household one by one turning unconscious sub and dominant pain and pleasure into correcting abject slaves' behaviour so they follow Christian living and do what the bible says. That's why I could never figure out who Jesus was as well as I was Jesus myself.

Last night's Journey now makes so much sense. When Meredith or should I say Real went to sleep I set about putting my plan into action. I told the whole world how I will put my plan of stopping the inevitable nuclear war into action... First I needed to check that Chorlton really was the head of world consciousness so I paraded through Hulme and Manchester University with my final preparations for the film of the century. Sophocles' Ancient Greek Tragedy being transformed into a modern film in the style of the 1979 classic The Warriors set in Hulme where the best graffiti in the country is.

I needed to go into the Classics Department itself. Make love to the girl I spoke to telepathically. Jane said it herself... When I told her about the film, as my dissertation. She said. "You really have everything sorted... I wish I could get my head as straight as yours Jason..." That was all the assurance I needed that I would have the right casting for the movie with my Classics team on board. Dr. Clarke and Dr Roy Gibson choosing the cast....

So next I walked through Mosside. Past, Denmark Road where I used to live. Worrying that I had killed that man I beat up who had tried to molest Meredith... I mean Mistress Real (visual manifestation in throne)... I set about visiting Mosside police station... I asked the officer: "is everything all right mate"... he said everything was and asked if I could help him with everything... I said of course I would and that I would be back. As I walked around Mosside trying to decide where the head of world consciousness was I came about more clues... First the old Bingo Hall run down. Nothing there sending spiritual messages that I was close. I went into a couple of newsagents and bought first the Caribbean Times and then an even more obscure ethnic minority newspaper. Very interesting but not quite the centre - it would be too obvious.

I'd been wondering all evening how it would happen and thought I would wait until Real was asleep to continue with the plan. As soon as she was asleep I sat on the empty gold fish bowl and made my seemingly submissive sexual ritual defecating in the bowl, filling it up with shampoo and then wrapping a plastic back around so the shit couldn't escape. I would present it to Real in the morning whilst it unconsciously made her my slave in her dreams. The next day when she discovered it she would assume that I was her slave and the role reversal and therefore the first steps to world peace would be underway.

In the evening I needed to send CHI in the opposite direction so first I took my Usual Suspects poster and placed it on the Garage on the house facing the right hand side of Cranbourne Road. Then I filled my rucksack with 30 or so significant literary texts, wrote cryptic messages to people I selected to spread the word and put them in every shop in Chorlton.

The fancy dress shops were of certain significance... that why I bought something for Real for everything during the afternoon... I can see why she was surprised when I gave them to her. All that flattery too much to bare for a mind that was still at times unconscious but I must not belittle her... such is the life and limits of a human being. It's difficult for me to remember now, as I have had the epiphany that the world has been waiting 2000 years for. It has hit me like a thunderbolt from Zeus.

The night certainly got more complicated and hectic as it grew on. My mind was racing like a Ferrari in a space shuttle. Had to remember what messages to send and where and how to present them so in the morning there would be only love in the air. That's why at 4.00am I thought I'd call Snoop Doggy Dogg and the Dogg Pound crew for help. I had Snoops number from the back of my Doggy Pound CD and went to a phone box to make the call. No one around... perfect. Pressing those numbers was like typing in the answers to the Universe. When I got to the other line I understood the coded message straight away. Snoop was on board and would spread the word to the record industry to put the live "All you need is Love" switch on as John Lennon and the Beatles had so publicly and quite charmingly enacted for me in the 60s. Then chance to join the physical and telepathic realms of the human race through sexual unconscious and conscious union where appropriate. A job well done and time to enjoy myself... and everyone else... ha ha ha...

Now I remember the next day when Meredith woke up not understanding the significance of the ritual.. the whole world on my shoulders... she took the day off work... it was affecting her life and set about taking me to see my mother in Wales. Fine by me.... Remember her imaginary role as the dominant was now crucial as part of this whole manoeuvring to stop the inevitable Nuclear War... Don't understand the logic... You're not meant to... too complex... only God can understand it... hence why I am retorting it right now...

I had some tasks to complete in the morning. To keep to schedule for when I had to be in the right place at the right time to discover time travel and shift between states I put on my roller skates and started giving banana's and cans of coke to the four tramps I saw that morning. I threw the significant book I'd saved up in the air at the garage.... Shouting the time is now... changed a few mindsets and thought patterns by being seemingly dangerous and crossing the road. Watched One Flew Over the Cuckoo's Nest as an Ode to the mentally ill in society and to put my telepathic judgement into all future Hollywood productions and creative ideas. During one scene of the film I swam under water to Australia and back again in less than five seconds. I had to try my reflexes for the pending rocket launch with my boogie board so on my back whilst stood in the living room. Real open the curtains (see Meredith opening curtains and Real's throne smiling – to different sides to the coin to explain one phenomenon) after her ecstasy was too much to bear and we were off to the train station via taxi.

After I bought a sports magazine to make get every famous sportsman, woman and team to start spreading the unconscious word of peace to all earth I met a charming lady on the train who reminded me of my Grandmother. Knowing she was the one who would understand I began giving her the details, coordinates and philosophy behind time travel. After forty five minutes I realised she had understood as Real had reassumed her earth mode as Meredith for a brief moment to suggest that I be quiet because she thought that the old lady had got "the idea by now". After a brief demonstration before leaving the train on showing time travel in action we set about reuniting with my mother…

This was very critical because Meredith back in her Real pose had made me realise that I needed to be in an isolated and anonymous place… i.e. out of the area where world consciousness was at its peak to enable the path to world peace and freedom to have the quickest effect. In the evening I telepathically made love to my mother and saw her as a matriarchal figure. I awoke in the middle of the night and stupidly told Meredith as I saw her for a split second that I needed help. "I knew I was manic and that I was desperately ill." Fortunately this thought subsided after a brief cry of some seven seconds and I was back into my plateau and god like state.

Could be an insert about reality of second episode and being in Talgarth – how about entrance and thinking I was film director upon arrival – mentioning of knife and game of pool before entering ?!

INTERNAL DIALOGUE 1: Fucking the Spice Girls scene.

Jason is sat down smoking a cigarette on a tiny, smelly and dirty hospital ward when out of the blue Professor Bain, a podgy late fifties man with grey hair, one of his lecturers, walks in.

JASON: Professor Bain. Surprised to see you hear. Thanks for visiting.

PROFESSOR BAIN: Ok. I was nosey, so here I am. Dr. Clarke sends his love.

Jason: That's nice.

PROFFESOR BAIN: I've bought you a book. It should be of real interest with your passion for films. Some light reading away from your final year studies. I hope it will be of interest.

JASON: The history of Hollywood. Thank you.

PROFESSOR: How are you?

JASON: Pretty terrible. I mean, I can see me getting through it. I'm not a quitter but it's the humiliation that's the worst thing. All those amazing thoughts that I thought I had were all rubbish. Not sure if I can ever come to terms with that.

PROFFESOR BAIN: Nodding his head. I see. You know we had a Professor who used to be in the department when I first started. Must be nearly thirty years ago now and he went mad like you. I came to see him in this hospital too. He got better and turned out to be one of the greatest classicists of our times. Most intelligent tutor we ever had in our department. The man was a genius. Graduated from Cambridge as I did.

JASON: Really - that's encouraging.

PROFFESOR BAIN: You're still young and have a good future ahead of you. Take this time to get some much needed rest. You will be back soon I presume.

JASON: I hope so. It will take me a month or two to recuperate.

PROFFESOR BAIN: Well I'll leave you and see you soon then. Dr. Clarke asks that you go and see him at the University when you feel up to it. I'll have him keep me informed of your progress.

JASON: Ok. Well thanks for coming.

PROFFESOR BAIN: Ok.

Dr. Clarke, a scruffy looking Irish intellectual in his late thirties is sat drinking a coffee with Jason in a quiet pub in Chorlton on a Sunday lunch time.

DR.CLARKE: Well Jason, it's very good to see you. I'm so pleased that you are better. You look good.

JASON: Thanks Dr. Clarke.

DR.CLARKE: Please call me Michael.

JASON: Ok sure.

DR.CLARKE: I'm sorry I didn't come to see you; I can't bear places like that. Something similar happened to me when I was younger, so I find it difficult to visit hospitals. Let's not talk about that though. Let's talk about you. How do you feel about returning this academic year?

JASON: I think it would be too difficult now. I've already missed the last seven weeks and my mood will drop before I get any better. It's how my manic cycles go.

Whenever I go high depression follows and it lasts even longer than the mania.

DR.CLARKE: Quite right Jason. I was going to advise you against it. You need time to heal and get better. Come back in the next academic year fresh and stronger. Then you'll stroll through the final year. You shouldn't give up on your degree and I'm sure you won't.

JASON: No I'll come back stronger. Will you still be there next year?

DR.CLARKE: Yes next year will be my last year in Manchester. Then I'm going back to Ireland to concentrate on writing my book.

JASON: What's the book about?

DR.CLARKE: The book is about gathering a collection of the finest war strategies from the Ancient Classical World. It will feature the most advanced strategies and the most epic battles in history including the most amazing victories against the odds.

JASON: Sounds fascinating.

DR.CLARKE: Yes, I've wanted to write it for some time now. Anyway, that's enough about me? How do you feel about everything?

JASON: I feel like I keep getting hit by the world's toughest boxer and it becomes increasingly more difficult to get back up.

DR.CLARKE: I thought you might say something like that. We all feel like that at one time or other. It's one of life's idiosyncrasies. Try and see it as a blessing in disguise. The harder you get hit by life the more you learn and the harder you are able to hit back. See life as a constant challenge. It would be boring if it was easy. I know you are going through great pain at the moment, but trust me that the most successful people in the history of this world are people who have suffered great hardship and uncertainty and managed to overcome it. Now you have experienced this manic depression again you have more potential to do greater good for yourself or even society if you want to. You could be a good example to many people if you want to. You have the ability to shape your own destiny and determine the way your own life turns out Jason. Remember that.

JASON: I will.

----

16 months later – final examination:

Final exam tripping out on Youth, Love and Rome 4 minutes:

INTERNAL DIALOGUE 1:

What is Lucan's own view on Civil War? Well Lucan is sick of it. He sees it as something that doesn't work. Why else would he be so obsessed with writing about it. Also he describe it in such grotesque detail that you could only feel that he was abhorrent. Just as the world feels abhorrent that I am a manic depressive but the truth is that Lucan must be fascinated by civil war as people are about my manic depression. I know that people are jealous of it and can explain my historical significance through the Classical World. Aeneas may have founded Troy but who founded the human race and invented the Greek and Roman Gods. I did and all unwittingly for my first twenty years. Strategically moving myself into position as a manic depressive in society's eyes so I could meet other like minded people who would remind me of my station.

I do not punish human beings for being above their station by giving them eternal madness like a Pentheus or an Ajax. I am not a Euripides or a Sophocles. I am too clever for that. That is why I created the most romantic story in the Ars Amatoria. Narcissus was punished it is true for being vain and the tragedy is that he will never see echo again because her voice, first voice, echoes so he will never know where to move. I myself although I know I am god, must not be overtly vain.

I must be humble so I am not guilty of 'hubrising' myself, a contradiction in terms I know but someone has to set the standards for the entire history of the universe. This brings me to my next point, about Catullus. He was in love with Lesbia we know and he was right about ancient Spanish people not cleaning their teeth. When he writes his poems it is fascinating to observe from a literary standpoint about the power of the in definability of being in the in crowd. For Catullus loves to join this crowd because it has no official size it is a matter of perception for him and in his poems he controls his own past.

In Ovid's Metamorphoses he appears to be sending a message of warning to the Emperor of the time Augustus saying how there will be a new Empire and a New Emperor that has its good and bad points. Ovid is really sending a message to me however. I created him as a writer to comment on the role of the Romans in history as part of the history of the world and made it a literary allusion to hide the obvious from the status quo, who would by nature cause anarchy if they knew everything. That would make my job twice as difficult and there has always been a lot to do as there is.... classics... manic energy... ancient rome... love... enjoy the manic feeling....

8 weeks later. October 1998.

Jason and his mum and dad are at Jason's Graduation on a sunny day outside the University. Jason is wearing his gown and hat and is posing for photos. Jason's mum and dad are both very proud whilst Jason is pumped full of medication.

MUM: Are you Ok dear?

Jason: Yeah. I feel stupid though with my eyes pumped full of this medication. Like my 18th birthday in Coney Hill. Remember that Mum. I was in hospital on my 18th birthday too and now my graduation.

MUM: looking upset. Oh dear. Come here.

DAD: Don't say that. You have done extremely well to make it considering what you have been through.

JASON: And what I've still got to go through.

DAD: I thought you said you knew why it happened?

MUM: Yes, overwork wasn't it.

JASON: …And binge drinking. Must stop that for good and with my psychologist I have ways of managing my stressors now so I know when my warning signs are and how to stop them.

DAD: Make sure you stop that drinking.

MUM: Sounds like you know what you are doing now dear. Don't try too hard. You always did try to run before you could walk you know. Ever since I can remember.

DAD: He's competitive like his dad. No harm in that.

MUM: No. No harm in being competitive, but everything doesn't need to happen all at once. Things take time.

JASON: I know. And this time I have strategies in place to cope with the boredom of the real world. I don't have a destructive personality any more and I know when to switch off. If things happen I'm going to switch off and when I deal with them I'll do so in a positive way.

MUM: Sounds like a personal transformation. Not heard you talk like that before Jay. Must be the pressure of University being over and everything, and that Psychologist has helped you, hasn't she. Kath, is that her name?

JASON: Yes, that's right she's set the scene but has told me that it is only me myself that can be the one who wants to get over this and manage it permanently in an effective manner.

DAD: Good - now stop waffling Jay and let's go in. Your ceremony begins in a few minutes. I want to get a good seat.

Jason collects his University Degree and his Mum and Dad are clapping in the audience.

July 1999. Jason is sat in the back garden on the floor in the sun reading the last page of the book Prozac Nation. When he finishes he closes the book smiles, looks up into the sky and says:

JASON: 'Right… let's do it…'

He goes into the house where the computer is already on and opens a word document. He then types 'A Can of Madness' by Jason Pegler into the page and then begins writing: 'how the fuck is someone meant to live with a mental illness? Don't ask me, still trying to find out how? After panning in and out of page of typing….. The doorbell rings. It is Gina, Jason's girlfriend at the time, and her friend Debbie.

Gina: "So have you started your thing a me jig yet?… You said you were going to when you finished that book….

JASON: Yes I've started it. It's going great. Want to see it?

GINA: Yeah. Let's go upstairs. Come on Deb. Race ya.

Jason sits by the computer and the girls sit on the bed.

GINA: Go on read it out then. You sexy writer, you!

JASON: Ok here it goes....

Jason reads out the first paragraph.... Gina interrupts I love the first line... I fucking love the first line.... 1 minute 30 second citation.....

Gina keeps screaming yes and jumps up and down on the bed. Then says she needs a cigarette. Debbie is already smoking and keeps shouting Yes...Yes.

GINA: You're onto a winner here. You're going to be famous. And it's so fucking true what you're saying. You're so right. Isn't that right Debs?

DEB: That's right Gene...

GINA: You know me and Debs have both been there and we know what its like. You sum it up man. You really sum it all up.

DEB: And you know what I really love about it Jason, is that you are being yourself. You still appear yourself in your writing. I know writers who completely change character when they put pen to paper and I don't usually mind that but I like the originality in this.

GINA: That's right original. So when are you going to buy me a brand new BMW then? How long will it be until you're famous? I bet you'll look real sexy in a nice shirt and tie on TV?

Jason talking sense will be able to see images of this speech and visually see the move to London as Renton moves to London in Trainspotting. This time music will be Coldplay with 'Clocks'.

JASON: I had to really choose life and move to London. That meant living the life that I wanted to. Having my third breakdown at the end of my University Degree had knocked back my confidence and I only stayed in Manchester and got a shitty job because my confidence had taken a knock again. I realised that I had to lead the life that I wanted to lead. That meant leaving Gina we'd both been moving in different directions. As soon as I started writing my autobiography I knew I'd finally find a cure. I was really on the road to recovery. All those years of anger and self fuelled resentment had been a waste of time. I wanted to focus on the very first realisation that I had when I returned to consciousness from my first manic episode. To psychoanalyse, myself and then set about helping reduce the humiliation of first one and then other sufferers where I could invent my own utopia to help mankind.

I moved to London to pursue a postgraduate fast track newspaper journalism course where it was cheap and moved in with a helpful landlord in Roger Moore's birthplace (play with James bond joke here) – the glamorous setting of Stockwell. Not paradise but a secure environment and next door to the college so very convenient. (Miami here or later?)Things were going well, then on the last day of college we had a university party and I met the love of my life. [Coldplay song becomes louder]. There is a beautiful moment of dancing, eye to eye contact and kissing with a beautiful Spanish girl with dark hair and big brown eyes. He takes her off the dance floor and asks her if she wants a coke. Her reply is "que?" We spent a few days together and felt spiritually very close.

There was a last holiday of destructive behaviour as if I needed to balance my whole life into perspective. I'd been given a free holiday to Miami thanks to (this bit filmed quickly like the guy slamming his drink down quickly in snatch hearing Benito Del Toro is off gambling) my landlord Felix, on the condition that I drive him around in a luxurious sports car to the odd business meeting. (Pan to driving red sports car.) There were two holidays in one. During the day I'd hang out with Felix going to the Everglades, watching Miami Heat, shopping, jet skiing on Christmas day and being shown sites by all the friendly people we met. When Felix crashed out any time from 10.30pm I'd be off binge drinking and cruising around in the sports car meeting people in bars and getting up to all sorts of mischief mainly drink driving and womanising. This culminated with a stupid occurrence where I mistakenly poured petrol into my eye at 9.00am when refuelling the car having been drink driving in between different bars without having any nights sleep.

After hitting 140 mph during the day and getting away with numerous traffic offences I set about turning home and pretty quickly settled into a relationship where I had one final episode in April 2000. By October 2000 I had recovered and finally got my own flat (show keys moving in,) thanks to the council. A bit run down but happy to do it up and get my life back on track the way it always should have been.

Psychologist Meeting: Summarising techniques

CAROL BUSCH: So Life is looking good, Jason, so how do you feel about everything?

JASON: I feel great. I have never felt so content about life, and the future looks good. More importantly I am enjoying every day.

CAROL BUSCH: Good for you Jason. How do you feel that the cognitive treatment has worked?

JASON: On the whole, I think the CBT has been great. I felt a bit uncomfortable at first letting my inner feelings out but after I soon felt comfortable talking about things with you. I think it is because that is the way it is designed. It feels that I am talking to you as a friend rather than a psychologist or part of the medical model and this makes things easier. The way we put together my action plan together was really a joint effort but a logical progression.

CAROL BUSCH: I'm so pleased Jason that you have found the treatment so helpful and you should congratulate yourself you have done well. You have put in a lot of hard work and deserve to be well. The action plan we put together was all your work. I was here to give you a structure of how to put your life into perspective and avoid stressors to reduce the risk of relapse and you worked with me very well. You know that you may come back and see me at any time should you ever feel the need to talk things over.

JASON: Thanks Carol. I know that but I think I'll be fine.

CAROL BUSCH: Well I hope so too Jason and I think you have a very good chance. You are a great deal better than when we first met and I feel that you've moved forward along way. Remember that this is not good bye however and that my offer still stands. All you need to do is ring the psychology department and speak to my secretary Grace. You know her don't you.

JASON: Yes I do. We know each other quite well now.

CAROL BUSCH: Good Jason. You know with the techniques you have learnt you have an excellent chance of staying well. I know that your work with your psychiatrist Dr Davies is equally important. How is that going along?

JASON: Well we are continuing to meet once every six weeks and the medication has kept me stable although I do intend to come off it for good in the near future.

CAROL: Well Jason I wish you luck. I must urge you not to come off your medication without discussing things with Dr. Davies. It really is most important.

JASON: Oh of course not, I will discuss any change in plan with him.

CAROL: Well I'm sure you will do Jason and I hope for your sake that you do. You have done extremely well and we want things to continue this way. If at any time you feel that I can be of any help whatsoever please do let me know. I am only a phone call away and whilst I am very busy, in fact busier than I have ever been, these days with the recent cut backs in the department should you need my help we would be able to meet within a few days.

JASON: Thanks Carol. I know you are and that is very reassuring. I am fine for now however and do not envisage us needing to see each other anymore on a regular basis. If at any time I need your help I will call you with no hesitation I promise.

CAROL: Ok...well thank you Jason.

JASON: Thank you Carol.

Meeting with DR. Davies about coming off medication but clearly more friendship here than anything else.

JASON: I know I am definitely Ok to come off the medication for good. I finally have the confidence to do it.

DR.DAVIES: I know you have really thought this through and you are doing very well.

JASON: I know you said that 90% of your patients relapse in the first year of coming off, but I know I have the strength of character to pull through especially with all these NLP techniques that I have learnt.

DR.DAVIES: Yes they sound very interesting. I feel that sometimes I could do with using some of the techniques you describe myself.

JASON: Well now you are my board with the charity I'll see if I can get you a free ticket to the world's greatest NLP practical trainer Anthony Robbins. Tickets are usually £455 but as a Chipmunka Foundation member maybe I can get you a free ticket, as long as you give me some feedback on how we could deliver this revolutionary practise to future NHS mental health patients.

DR.DAVIES: Why I'd be delighted.

JASON: I am more myself now than I have been for a long time, since I was seventeen probably and now I am on a lower dose of medication – 600mg of Sodium Valporate a day I can see the side effects of the drug. It blocks my real feelings, makes me anxious and confused. The sooner I am off them the better but I am happy to come off them gradually over the next three months like you said.

DR.DAVIES: Yes coming off gradually is wise.

JASON: And I know I can take my sleeping tablets if I need them. When should I take them?

DR.DAVIES: Well you need at least four hours of sleep a night. Ideally you should have about 7.00 but some people can manage with less. If you cannot sleep the first night take your sleeping pill the next night. Start with one.

JASON: If I still can't sleep what should I do? Can I take up to 4 3.5mg of Zopiclone in a night.

DR.DAVIES: Yes no more than that and try to take less than that.

JASON: What next?

DR.DAVIES: If you still have trouble sleeping on the fifth day, go onto 50mg of Zopiclone like we talked about. That should calm you down. Then once you have had a good few days of sleep you can come off it.

JASON: Yes I remember. It's better to have to go on a stronger drug the Quetiapine for a few days and suffer the more serious side effects from that than endure the side effects of the Sodium Valporate all of the time.

DR.DAVIES: Yes that's right.

JASON: I don't envisage needing to do this though but I will be honest with myself if at any time I definitely need to. I am so much better at managing my life now and things are going really well with my work. Chipmunka is going really well. We've been in all the national newspapers and I've been on TV several times lately and been invited to the States to appear on TV and talk as well.

DR.DAVIES: Yes I hear from some of my colleagues that you are doing extremely well. I am very pleased. Your work is helping a lot of people I am sure and I am proud that you have asked me to be a part of it.

JASON: Well, like I said on TV the other week, it is vitally important to have a psychiatrist that treats you as a human being first and not a patient. Only then can you build up a rapport and start to help the patient to help themselves.

DR.DAVIES: That makes a lot of sense to me... Well time is running a little short. Let's make our next appointment in three weeks time so we can monitor how you feel as you reduce the dosage...ok?

JASON: Ok, let's do this.

Dr. Davies leads Jason out of the room. He opens a security door and they go into the waiting room.

DR.DAVIES: Please can you give Jason another appointment. [Addressing the Chinese male 20ish receptionist in the window]

RECEPTIONIST: Looks at the diary. When would you like it?

DR.DAVIES: 3 weeks time please?

RECEPTIONIST: How about Friday the 19th?

JASON: That's fine.

RECEPTIONIST: I'll put it in my diary.

DR.DAVIES: Well Jason... [Shaking hands] I look forward to seeing you soon. Take care.

JASON: Yes, and you chief. Take care. Bye.

Richard and Judy interview:

JUDY: And now to a truly remarkable story

RICHARD: Yes, we are extremely lucky to have him here. Believe me all of us are.

JUDY: Yes, Richard I agree entirely. Here he is, the Founder of Chipmunkapublishing and the Chipmunka Foundation, and of course the author of the world's most significant book on mental illness. Jason Pegler.

Jason walks in with a casual grey suit and T-shirt on. Shakes Richard's hand smiling and kisses Judy who wipes a tear away from here eye.

RICHARD: Allow me to start, if I may Jason. Your selfless work is quickly becoming recognised as a force for social good, most notably reducing stigma on mental health by so cleverly creating the world's first mental health brand. I have one question though, which I am sure you are often asked but I am fascinated to know. Why did you feel so compelled to write A Can of Madness? It can't have been an easy decision. What made you do it?

JASON: Well Richard, it's quite simple. It came to me in a flash. When I was seventeen I'd been in a mental hospital for six weeks and I thought I'd been playing Football Manager, the computer game. The moment I realised where I was, I knew that the only way I could ever psychoanalyse myself and emotionally get over the humiliation that I felt was to tell the whole world how I felt, and create a Hollywood blockbuster movie about my experiences. I knew that deep down I had the mental strength to do this and I knew I had a responsibility to stop the humiliation that anyone else who has ever been in a mental hospital feels.

JUDY: I'm so pleased, and I know Richard is too, to have you on the show. Please explain to us in more detail and to the viewers at home, what you mean by humiliation and give us an idea what drives you.

JASON: Of course Judy. Let me explain it like this. The moment I realised I was in a mental institution I felt guilty, humiliated for having a mental illness and I knew that this was something that was fundamentally wrong. It was society that made me and makes anyone with mental health issues feel like this. Thing is that we are all so close to it really. Having manic depression myself changed me as a person, made me more sensitive and gave me insight as a human being that I would not have had otherwise. In fifty years time, when another seventeen year old is in the same position as me, the moment he realises, the first thought that will go through his mind will be "I'm manic and society is going to help me" not "I'm manic and its my fault, I'm a freak" . Then I've made a happy man. That is what drives me every day and why I do what I do.

RICHARD: I see Jason…so, let's look at the present - you are the head of The Chipmunka Group and creator of the World's First Mental Health Brand. What's next?

JASON: Well Richard, to continue with the mission and release 'A Can of Madness' as the Hollywood Blockbuster Movie I always intended it to be. I must stress that this is for the benefit of society. It is beyond my own ego. I have maintained the IPR and creative direction so that I can keep the story real and grow the brand through philanthropic activity. The World is badly managed and to eliminate mental ill health and psychiatry for good we need to be focused. We can't afford to waste time, as people's lives are at stake.

RICHARD: I have heard rumours that Tom Cruise will be starring in the film Jason, is that true?

JASON: Let's just say that I know someone who is close to Tom's heart and I think it would be a wonderful project for him. He is such a wonderful actor and his films are very influential.

JUDY: Well I know I'm definitely going to see it. I would like to refer to psychiatry though, if I may? I mean, it's pretty radical what you're saying don't you think?

JASON: Well it's more common sense Judy, actually. Let me explain it like this. Psychiatry was invented as a form of social control. If people behave oddly, there has to be rules put in place otherwise there would be anarchy. Then look at the history of schizophrenia, for example. In 1908 some Suisse scientist advertised a notice locally asking who heard voices. Several people came forward. Some enjoyed their voices whilst it disturbed others. The scientist then calls this schizophrenia and then some entrepreneur, not a social one I hasten to add, thinks 'I know. I'll sell some drugs and make a fortune'. That's how it happens. And the whole world is taught to think that we need these drugs that screw our minds up.

I've seen hundreds of thousands of people better off without them, myself included. All that's needed is a positive that is reinforced on a daily basis and you'll never need to suffer the horrid side effects of any psychiatric drugs.

RICHARD: Yes I know people to who you have helped who have been well for years after reading your book and hearing you and Chipmunkapublishing authors speak. That is why I am so delighted that you could spare the time for us to appear on this show.

JUDY: Yes Jason. Mental health is a subject that is so very close to my heart.

JASON: Thanks to both of you. I'd just like to remind the audience at home that you must do something today to help the mental health of someone else. Give love back and it will return tenfold.

RICHARD: Oh I nearly forgot to say congratulations on winning the New Statesman's Young Social Entrepreneur of the Year Award 2005.

JASON: Thank you.

JUDY: I hear you beat Jamie Oliver in the process. You must be proud.

JASON: It means so much to receive the recognition not for my own ego but because it shows that the judges realised the vitally important work that we are doing. There is so much good will out there and we have a duty to maximise it for the benefit of everyone.

On the beach front on a Sunny morning 6.30am in Barcelona.

JASON: "Ah finally finished. At last the script to change the way Hollywood and the world thinks about mental health once and for all and the deal is already signed. Think I'll have a shower".

SONIA: "Ok sweetie. Well done".

JASON: "Thanks sweetie".

SONIA: "How did you manage to do it so quickly?"

JASON: I managed to focus as you know, exercise every morning, wrote what was in my heart and stayed true to myself. All the time, I envisioned that it was already completed in the way that I wanted it to be. There was a burning desire within me to complete it because I know that when it is out it will help people who watch it and are influenced by the world's reaction to it.

SONIA: "I see" smiling.

STEPHEN SPIELBERG: Jason that's great. Next take remember just be yourself. You've experienced this before so all you are doing is reliving it.

JASON – talking to the actor playing the character of his English teacher in the school and the film set.

JASON: "I have taken 5 billion ecstasy tablets, one for everyone on earth to create world peace, so I can fulfil my obligations as Head of the European hardcore Committee and instil love as one family."

PAMELA: How realistic do you think this is? You are not well.

JASON: Do not worry about me. Where there is a will there is a way. I only wish that you could see what I see... Think of those hardcore lyrics Miss... Into the future. We'll live as one family... They were written for a reason and I have discovered the reason... I have it all mapped out in front of me... look at my action plan... I will control Hollywood and the way it thinks by planting subliminal messages of peace onto the world... this is so exciting to have found the answer.. Then I can get my message out... I'll use telepathy to raise the consciousness of people around me to get them to unwittingly buy into this ideal... the world is our oyster...

PAMELA: What do your parents say about all of this?

JASON: They don't understand yet but they are starting to.

PAMELA: I think you need some help Jason.

JASON: I know. That's why I am here. Don't worry - we can do this.

They hold hands for a moment. Pamela is crying feeling desperately upset as she sees Jason as needing urgent help. Jason holds Pamela's hands thinking he is telepathically in tune with womankind to create world peace through the European Hardcore Committee which he set up as a means of communication from heaven and the real world.

Jason drives along Hollywood Boulevard in his red Ferrari listening to 2 Pac's California Love. He gets out of the car and walks into a very nice restaurant. As he is invited to sit down by the waiter Jack Nicholson stands up.

JACK: How's it going kids?

JASON: "Going great, thanks Jack. Jack how are you?
JACK: Not so bad. The Nicks won so I'm happy. You know I really think you're going to win the Oscar with "A Can of Madness this Year". I've not been as excited since "One Flew Over the Cuckoo's Nest was at this stage, just a week away from the result.

JASON: Wow thanks Jack.

JACK: You see... you got guts kid. Not only did you write the script but you acted in it and had a hand in the direction as well. You kept the story real...you see what I'm saying?

JASON: Yes Jack. I've spent years planning this. I just hope it happens. Not for my sake but for the sake of people's mental health. If it wins the Oscar next week in February 2007 then this adds recognition forever in Hollywood. It means that the taboo of mental health will disappear once and for all and then it will be easier to help the third world achieve Equal Lives.

JACK: Right on. What you having to eat. I'll have the salad. How about you?

JASON: Same here and a raw juice.

JACK: Sounds great. I'll have one too. Now tell me about your next film.

JASON: Well it's another autobiography about mental health. This one is just as inspiring...

JACK: Now why did I think that?

JASON: Well it comes from this utopian vision of wanting to stop the humiliation of anyone who has ever had a mental health issue. It concerns setting up a generation of people to come forward and be positive about their past pains so they can empower themselves and other people. There are different social and financial systems in place.

Imagine the world as the planet Saturn and in the middle is the ring the mission to stop the humiliation of everyone. At the top is an arrow pointing down. Mental Well-being leading down to mental illness. The mental well being model reached to reduce stigma and vice versa. The more people are proactive in reducing stigma the further up the planet people go. The more people look after their own mental well being i.e. Mind, Body and Soul, the more time they will have to help a person with a mental health issue empower themselves.

Take the same scenario with a financial model. At the top you have a philanthropic model sending money the right way for the right reasons for this utopian ideal. At the bottom you have charity and social enterprise models campaigning in proactive terms. They have influence and can create good will but do not change the world as a whole.

JACK: – I see. Marvellous.

JASON: Well I better stop there because that's a manic mind after all and I want to eat.... hey, listen Jack... I love this song.

Coldplay's "clocks" starts playing in the background and continues through the credits.

Panning out of vision like beginning of Star Wars i.e. some mental health facts... or map of Saturn diagram... but has serious undertone and plays with screen like beginning of Amelie.

Chapter Eight

Conclusion: "Curing Madness, The end of Madness – the beginning of equilibrium and a fair world"

It is inevitable that madness on earth as we know it will end. Too many people have suffered for too long. Since the beginning of time people who are the weakest have been eliminated or humiliated. Eventually they will join forces and create a bond that will lead to a revolution. I am talking about the plight of the "mentally ill". During this philosophical treatise I will prove that everyone on earth has a mental health problem.

I will begin with the strongest philosophical argument to date. That is that madness is a social construct i.e. it has been created by the status quo as a means of social control. In fact according to American Professor John Breeding, psychiatry is the greatest form of social control since Hitler and his anti Semitism in the Second World War. Breeding's argument is very impressive and is explained in layman terms, so a wide audience can be reached, but we must delve deeper.

I myself, for example, agree with Breeding's wonderful argument but as a manic depressive since the age of seventeen I have been unable to escape the social construct that I am a part of. I cannot go and live on another planet in a world where prejudice, stigma and no humiliation or even hubris exists, as I have the limits of being a human being. This leaves me with manic depression, in the real world, even though I know that it fundamentally doesn't exist. My mind though, is able to wander through in NLP mode and envisage a utopian ideal, where a positive image of mental health, developed by the mental health service users themselves, can lead to a revolution whereby the world is cured of mental illness. I can therefore visualise or incant a cure and choose to stay in these preferable states of being.

The utopian ideal is as follows. If I can prove that everyone on earth has a mental illness then I can stop the humiliation that mental health sufferers go through and ultimately improve that madness is after all merely a social construct. If this can be achieved then we will be able to break down mental health as a taboo and normalise it so that is mainstream an integral to society. Once it is integral to society people will have owned up and then admit to each other their own vulnerabilities. This creates a caring culture instead of a punitive one and leads to the empowerment of the mental health service user.

A most poignant example is Martin Luther King JNR and black rights in the 1960s. Thank the world for Rosa Parks who inspired Martin Luther King and countless others. If Martin Luther King JNR was a white person talking about black people's experiences nobody would have listened to him. The fact that he led a peaceful demonstration is also significant. Promoting a positive image on mental health is also a key factor in making the masses and government's buy into the strategy and have the empathy that is desired by so many sufferers. The mental health sufferer must be seen in an over positive light. This is to compensate for the disadvantageous way they are represented by the media, in flippant conversations and by the people who care for them when they are in their worst or most creative states.

We currently understand mental illness as a disease because governments, drug companies and psychiatry tell us so. However, as Breeding and Thomas SSAS and so eloquently put it, let's look at the "facts" as they are laid out in front of us. Only once we have done this, can we see how we as a world can join together and look after the well being of each other so there is no longer any need for people to experience mental illness whatever it may or may not be.

The future of mental health empowerment, the world's first mental health brand and in my view the solution to curing my own madness of and the world which i perceive and am therefore part of is very simple.

It lies in the hands of the people. It was never designed to be owned by an individual, just representatives, who by positively discriminating in their own favour, could plant the seeds for a social revolution across the globe. Chipmunka is driven by empowerment, for the people of the world to stop the ultimate humiliation in life. That is of being diagnosed with a metaphor that turns into a poisonous reality, unless the pattern is broken and creativity and humanity are allowed to flow, and raise one's consciousness and standards back to reality.

Whatever you believe you are entitled to. That is your right as an individual. I wrote this book to illustrate how i cured myself and to give love to other people in the world who have been severely damaged by mental illness. I wanted to reveal the truth about my own experiences and to show others that you too can cure yourselves if you want to. This is because i honestly believe that there deep down there is nothing wrong with you. Insanity and mental illness are merely a matter of perception at the end of the day.

If anyone tells you any different they either have vested interests, are self manifesting their own mental illness or fear change. If we all visualise a world without mental illness then it will cease to exist in other people's realities and as a social construct. This is a matter of fact so lets do it. That is how i transformed myself and that is why i have dedicated my life to helping others see this opportunity to embrace life and achieve the impossible by saying no to a life of mental illness. I keep doing this by growing my inner self every day and being in a constant state of creative being. Now it's your turn. Enjoy it and please do keep in touch.

There is of course amazing work done by mental health charities around the world that have been campaigning for generations to help people in mental distress. I want to acknowledge all of their hard work and let them know that all of us involved with the Chipmunka Group and the many wonderful mental health groups around the world will endeavour to work with people who have had difficult times and help them to help us all to take further steps in improving the well being of the planet. Giving back is what really excites me as we all make the transition from mental illness to mental well being.